LIVING WITHOUT AIDS

Helping families and youth win the fight against AIDS and attaining a new dimension of exceptional living

Oladipo Obisesan

Together We Can Exterminate AIDS
"Everything is possible"

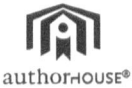

authorHOUSE®

This book is available at special quantity discounts for bulk purchase for sales promotions, premiums, groups, fund-raising, and educational needs. For details, write AuthorHouse, 500 Avebury Boulevard, Central Milton Keynes, MK9 2BE, or telephone 08001974150.

AuthorHouse™ UK Ltd.
500 Avebury Boulevard
Central Milton Keynes, MK9 2BE
www.authorhouse.co.uk
Phone: 08001974150

Published in association with:
Dipo Obisesan Prayer Ministries and Living Without AIDS Mission
www.dipoobisesan.com
www.livingwithoutaids.com

First published by AuthorHouse   3/26/2010

ISBN: 978-1-4490-8406-6 (sc)
ISBN: 978-1-4520-0653-6 (dj)

This book is printed on acid-free paper.

Printed in the United States of America Bloomington, Indiana

Although I have known Oladipo Obisesan only a short time, I have seen his integrity and devotion to the Lord through his writing and through our communication. He writes with a godly passion to a world in which immorality is rampant. Even so, writing from a Christian perspective, Dipo (as I've come to know him) gives hope to a hurting world where millions face the challenge of dealing with one of the products of this immorality—HIV/AIDS.

In his book, *Living without AIDS*, Oladipo is straightforward in dealing with this worldwide problem. He clearly shows the history, the medical aspects, and the causes of this dread disease. But he doesn't stop there. One thing I like most about this book is that it is not full of condemnation but rather full of compassion, which I believe the church can learn from.

The author is highly qualified to write on the subject and writes from a Biblical perspective. You as the reader will be informed and enriched by the store of knowledge that Oladipo brings to the page.

-B. Kay Coulter

Editor for The Write Way Editorial Services

Author of *Proverbs for Personalities,*
Victim/Victor: It's Your Choice, and *Free to Be*

Temple, Texas

During the editing of this book, I have come to know it well and have gained a great respect for the sincerity and dedication with which the author is fulfilling his divine mission to educate people on the facts about HIV/AIDS and the need to live a life that reflects morality and compassion. I have dedicated much of my own time to helping him deliver this message because his words have touched my heart and I share his wish that they reach as wide an audience as possible.

When I accept a manuscript for editing, I never know quite where it may lead me. The same is true for the book you hold in your hand. My work is now complete, and I am proud to call Oladipo Obisesan my good friend. We come from different parts of the world and different spiritual points of view, yet his work has inspired me, and I believe it will be inspiring to many others.

Living without AIDS is written from a Christian perspective, but the messages are universal. If you do not happen to be of the Christian persuasion, you can easily understand his message as applying to your own belief in a Creator, for the One God is the God of us all. No matter how we think of that Supreme Power, we can pray for a cure and do all in our limited power to establish our lives and the lives of our children on deeply held moral convictions. This is what is needed to effect a lasting global solution to the terrors of HIV/AIDS.

And what are those desired moral convictions? They have been put forward by every great religion of the world: treating our neighbors as ourselves and also treating ourselves with the same consideration we would extend to a loved one, cultivating kindness and compassion, believing in the richness of our truly human capacity, living according to standards of decency, not engaging in or tempting through our habits behavior that is risky, and knowing that principles of right living have been extolled throughout the ages for our own good. The people of the Bible were asked to refrain from unrestrained sexuality and infidelity and to adhere to habits of clean living for a reason: when they ignored God's commands, these behaviors unnecessarily exposed them to *wasting disease* and untimely death. Today, also, we can see that there are grave risks associated with immoral behavior, and when we take unnecessary risks, we are gambling with our lives.

Many HIV-positive people are walking around unaware of their HIV status and the help that they could receive. You cannot look in the mirror and know whether you have been infected with HIV. You cannot look at another person and know whether he or she is HIV-positive. This is why you must always take precautions, and abstinence outside of marriage and a faithful marriage are the only guarantees for living without AIDS.

With great compassion, the author makes it clear that, if you live a moral life, you do not need to be afraid. People with AIDS need friendship, understanding, and affection, and you cannot contract HIV by hugging them or even by eating off the same plate. Our tendency to shun those who are afflicted only increases the spread of AIDS by making people fear testing. It may seem easier not to know. However, early detection can make the difference between life and death. You can live a long life as an HIV-positive person if you detect the disease early and get the proper medical treatment.

In addition to knowledge and understanding about AIDS, I was enriched by the author's message about the power of prayer and the hope offered by a positive attitude toward life. I was particularly struck by these words: *"I know that I have everything I want, because if I really wanted it, I know that my Lord would provide it for me."* In my own life at the time, and now, I am reminded to ask God for what I need. We were not meant to have lives filled with hardship. God has bestowed on each of us a special gift that we can discover and fulfill, and through that gift we can benefit others and receive everything we need. I have no need—ever—to be discouraged.

And so, when I am downhearted or discouraged, I will remember this book and my friend. I hope, like me, you will never forget these words of Scripture that the author quotes so frequently: "Everything is possible." Yes, it truly is. Even a world without AIDS is possible.

-Sarah Risko Aschenbach

Editor and Author

Relationships Made Easy: How to get along with all kinds of people

Coatesville, PA

IMPORTANT NOTE

This book is written in simple terms in order to communicate life-saving information to the family and it is intended to supplement personal medical advice from medical professionals to patients and to educate anyone who wishes to understand more about HIV/AIDS, but it is not a substitute for such advice.

You should also note that advanced medical research to defeat AIDS is ongoing and A CURE will be found in the not too distant future. You are, however, strongly advised not to take any medication unless you have gone through a blood test to enable your medical doctor to discover your status and give the necessary treatment your personal situation demands. With God, "everything is possible."[1] Yes, it is. A permanent cure for AIDS is possible.

Before undergoing any medical treatment,
**YOU SHOULD ALWAYS CONSULT YOUR
MEDICAL PROFESSIONAL.**

More than 25 million people have died of AIDS since 1981.

Africa has over 14 million AIDS orphans.

At the end of 2008, women accounted for 50% of all adults living with HIV worldwide

In developing and transitional countries, 9.5 million people are in immediate need of life-saving AIDS drugs; of these, only 4 million (42%) are receiving the drugs. Sources: UNAIDS (2009, November), "AIDS epidemic update."

DEDICATION

"A father of the fatherless, a defender of widows, is God in His holy habitation"

For all the children and women all over the world who have been orphaned by HIV/AIDS and for those who are currently living with HIV/AIDS. Christ said that He would not leave you to be orphans; He will come to you. The Comforter alone can comfort you if you allow Him to dwell with you and be in you. I say *Hakuna Matata*: don't worry. Just hold on and do not give up. Help has come.

CONTENTS

ACKNOWLEDGMENTS

He raises the poor from the dust
And lifts the beggar from the ash heap,
To set them among princes
And make them inherit the throne of glory.
"For the pillars of the earth are the LORD'S,
And He has set the world upon them.
He will guard the feet of His saints,
But the wicked shall be silent in darkness.
"For by strength no man shall prevail."
(1 Samuel 2:8 NKJV)

I remember when I came to the city of Lagos as a village boy who could barely talk in the midst of friends and colleagues. Today, I acknowledge how the Word of the Lord and the Holy Spirit have transformed me from a life of inferiority complex to a life of audacity. I had intended to write a pamphlet, but divine inspiration transformed the pamphlet into a masterpiece. O Lord, I thank You at this defining moment in history, for You have done what the skeptics thought we could not do. By God's special favor and mighty power, I have been given the wonderful privilege to author a book on this important subject, HIV/AIDS (wasting disease), although I did nothing to deserve it, and this has been absolutely beyond my control. The Holy Spirit did it, and for this cause, I bow my knees to the Father of our Lord Jesus Christ, the Creator of everything in heaven and on earth, and I say thank You for Your abundant provision for this mission. From Your glorious and unlimited resources, You gave me mighty inner strength through Your Holy Spirit. I am forever grateful to the Father of our Lord Jesus Christ. It took years to write this book, but divine inspiration does not expire. Grace be with those who love our Lord Jesus Christ in sincerity. Amen

I sincerely recognize the brotherly love, humility, and meekness of my spiritual father, Pastor Ayo Daniels. You took me by the hand and encouraged me so much on this mission. God will extend this great kindness to your own children.

My spiritual grandfathers Pastor E.A Adeboye, Pastor W.F Kumuyi, Dr. David Oyedepo, and Pastor Sam Adeyemi, your exceptional teaching has helped transform my spiritual life.

I acknowledge the good effort of the forty-third president of the United States, George W. Bush, who while in office launched the President's Emergency Plan for AIDS Relief, also known as PEPFAR, which is America's initiative to combat the global HIV/AIDS epidemic. This global initiative has spared millions of lives.

I am very grateful to Olusegun Peleyeju (Ph.D.), whom God used to structure this book; and others like Pastor Kayode Akosile, Pastor Taiwo Dixon, Pastor Yinka Adesanya, Rev. Deborah Odutola, Pastor and Mrs. Radex Oluwatimilehin, Pastor and Mrs. Sola Olatunji and Pastor Omoyele Mary Afolabi.

I bestow this honor upon my late mother, Omokeinde Obisesan, who wanted me to become a medical doctor, and upon my late father, Chief Samuel Oyewole Obisesan, who wanted me to become a policeman like he was. Both my parents wanted me to serve humanity in different capacities. Today, your dreams for me have been fulfilled because my Creator, God Almighty, has enlisted me in His army, and that has enabled me to serve humanity in a bigger and better capacity. Glory and honor to the Hope of Glory.

With sincerity of heart, I thank Princess Ifedolapo Tinuala. God bless you for your patience and love. Your value cannot be measured by any standard. You are more than a champion. Thank you for being my support and encourager.

In life there are friends, but God blessed me with great friends like Ojediran Stephen, Sola and Keinde Oguntunde, Dr. Solape and Fade Adegbehingbe, Toyin Deinde, Deji Fatiregun (Ph.D.), Tunji Adeleye, Wole Jaiyeola, Eddy Aina, Femi Olurinola, Bisola Olabode, Ayo Omobgemi, Ayo Irale and other exceptional friends.

Special thanks go to Sarah Risko Aschenbach, my editor. God used you to edit this book. Your editing is outstanding. I appreciate your friendship, commitment, and skill. I am proud to call you an excellent editor.

I greatly appreciate the extraordinary commitment and enthusiasm of Brenda K. Coulter, who provided key editorial assistance as well as valuable Biblical insights and perspectives. Kay, I am proud to know you.

I am happy to extend my profound gratitude to all the Ninth Hour companions. Thank you for believing in God's vision.

This divine inspiration creates divine aspiration, and now we have a book called *Living without AIDS*. Truly, with God on our side, *everything is possible*. Yes, it is.

"It is difficult to imagine how the world can grow together and overcome the instabilities and inequalities of global interdependence unless something serious is done to turn the tide on AIDS"

-President Bill Clinton

PROLOGUE

The first thing is character . . . Money cannot buy it . . . because a man I do not trust could not get money from me on all the bonds in Christendom. — *J.P.Morgan[2]*

In my great country, Nigeria (*Good People, Great Nation*), it is required to undergo one year of national service after university education, and as I was rendering this service to my great country, I received the inspiration to write this book. I realized that HIV/AIDS was a battle that must be won within the family. This realization created a burden in my spirit. As I sat down one afternoon in my office gazing at my computer and thinking on the fact that youths in remote environments might not have access to a life-saving information on AIDS, it settled strongly on my spirit to a least produce a pamphlet that can be distributed to those in remote areas. I further told one of my co-coordinators at work, Mrs. Nkechi Mordi, that as soon as I get a paying job, I will be using ten percent of my monthly salary for this purpose. The result of my thinking eventually generated a clear vision to save this generation and the next from HIV/AIDS, which is perhaps the most dreadful disease in the world today. Its unprecedented spread across different countries of the world within the past few years evokes fear in the minds of all that the human race may possibly face extinction within a short while unless appropriate measures are taken. If we all can come together, this trend is reversible, and the vision of overcoming the HIV/AIDS scourge is achievable by the grace of God. Together, we can exterminate AIDS. I believe, as the Scripture promises, "Everything is possible."

AIDS, an acronym for Acquired Immunodeficiency Syndrome, and its precursor HIV (Human Immunodeficiency Virus) develops when an individual has blood contact with someone already infected with the virus. This can happen through sexual activities, blood transfusion, childbirth, the sharing of sharp objects, and through other means that this book will enunciate.

HIV/AIDS now resides in our conservative environment, in which people do not openly discuss their health issues. Our significant weapons to fight the scourge in the home, in the workplace, and on the street are knowledge and a thorough understanding: first, that AIDS is real; and second, that there is presently NO CURE; and finally, that acquisition of WISDOM for the fight begins with every individual.

Knowledge = Understanding = Wisdom

Knowledge brings awareness; it delivers the information about HIV/AIDS to you. Knowledge is what you will acquire by reading this book. Thus, the saying that knowledge is potential power is absolutely correct.

In turning the tide against HIV/AIDS, understanding is the key to living without it. Understanding is a significant step after knowledge. Knowledge conveys information, but understanding unravels the mystery behind it. Knowledge is narrowed to what you can see, hear, and read, but thorough understanding helps you acquire the wisdom necessary for actualizing what you have acquired via knowledge. Understanding comes when you ask yourself questions such as: "How can I avoid HIV/AIDS?" and "Why is it that HIV/AIDS may not be readily apparent?" Upon obtaining answers to these questions, you must process your knowledge of the disease into understanding through the use of applied reasoning and meditation. When you follow these steps, wisdom comes in and helps you do what must be done. Wisdom is a force that motivates you to act meticulously. It brings you full knowledge and understanding. Wisdom tells you that abstinence remains your best viable option for avoiding HIV/AIDS. Along with exercising due care in refraining from sharing sharp objects, wisdom also tells you to break out of every relationship that introduces sex as a prerequisite for intimacy or marriage. Do not be fooled into keeping wrong friends, since bad company corrupts good character.

In the course of my service, my experience with teenagers revealed that, although they are the most vulnerable to HIV/AIDS, they lack core moral values and life-saving information about the disease. Those who are very knowledgeable about it but lack understanding play down the disease and make it appear less serious than it really is. As I have said, understanding of HIV/AIDS is crucial to avoiding the disease. The teenagers I encountered lacked moral education and good understanding, which are needed if you want to live without the disease. Everyone needs more than mere knowledge about HIV/AIDS. We need to realize that knowledge and understanding of HIV/AIDS complement each other.

This, consequently, has given me the resolve to write on the relationship between human blood, HIV/AIDS (wasting diseases), and moral character, the latter of which is mostly lacking in the life of today's youth. Blood, especially the white blood cells, energizes the body's system to fight diseases. HIV gradually breaks down these cells. Moral uprightness, on the other hand, creates a barrier that prevents entry of HIV.

HIV is not a contagious disease; sexual immorality is one of the vehicles it uses to penetrate the blood. An insight into this relationship will enhance your knowledge and understanding of the scourge. During Biblical times, lack of moral character destroyed the entire family of Lot, Abraham's nephew, and killed twenty-three thousand people the day after they acquired wasting diseases through acts of sexual immorality.

Today, lack of moral character in the family and society in general has caused many to acquire HIV, and millions of people have died from AIDS. We can avoid or prevent wasting disease, which is synonymous with AIDS, if our characters are rooted in core moral values and uprightness. What the world lacks is not money or technology, but core moral standards, which are significantly missing in every nation around the world. The principal value is character. Money does not produce character, but money flows in the direction of a man with good character.

In turning the tide against AIDS, understanding is the key.

If moral uprightness can prevent indecent practices and, consequently, HIV, then in today's world, what our children need most are not thousands of shares of stocks, but guided moral character. In the words of Scripture, "Riches will not help on the day of judgment, but right living is a safeguard against death."[3] They also say, "Upright citizens are good for a city and make it prosper but the talk of the wicked tears it apart."[4] Right living, and not money, is what will save our children from HIV/AIDS. Right-living people are the richest individuals in terms of blessings, integrity, honor, dignity, kindness, and wisdom. The integrity of the upright shall guide them into tremendous success. Therefore, guided morals will deliver the best future into our children's hands, because once they have righteous principles, they will not fail to perform virtuous actions. Virtue is neither genetic nor inborn; it is the positive sign of moral uprightness and the nobility of a soul.

Readers of all ages will find this book indispensable. It offers sensible and practical suggestions on how to manage the disease, relate with those already infected and, best of all, avoid being a victim of HIV/AIDS. The book is directed at adding value to your life, making you think, and changing your mindset against people living with HIV/AIDS. It will give you the sufficient understanding you need to protect yourself, your family and friends.

I hope this book will truly fulfill the task for which it is intended. *Use this book to improve your understanding of HIV/AIDS, but if you are already a victim, do not delay in seeking medical assistance.* Let the awareness about this pandemic increase! Let our youth put sex on hold and seek knowledge about HIV, and let them live their lives based on core moral standards, which are kingdom principles. My hope is that this book will be the springboard to a life of moral excellence and one free of HIV/AIDS.

**A sick soul needs knowledge, because knowledge
and its proper use can win the battle against HIV/AIDS.**

May the beauty of the Lord, our God, be upon you, establish your success, and give you rapid understanding as you settle down to a voyage of discovery. A world without AIDS is possible. *With God, everything is possible.* Yes, it is.

CHAPTER ONE
HISTORICAL ACCOUNT OF
THE KILLER DISEASE

*What has been is what will be and what has been done is what will be
done: there is nothing new under the sun. Can one say about anything
"Look, this is new"? It has already existed in the ages before us.*[1]

The Bible, which is an authority over history, accounted that
nothing—physical, philosophical, scientific, or artistic—is absolutely
new under the sun. There may be many discoveries as God increases
human wisdom, but all things have their origins in the ages preceding
us. Because God's Word has come down as wisdom to all the genera-
tions, it is about time we look profoundly into the Word of God, which
has authority over all things, to ascertain the origin and source of this
deadly disease, HIV/AIDS.

From the inception of HIV/AIDS, humans have put as much effort
as possible into trying to establish its origin and source. Even so, we
have not been able to specifically or logically ascertain that origin and
source. The history of this epidemic might just be what was accounted
for in the Sacred Book, which said that between 1450–1410 B.C., the
act of sexual immorality paved the way for the acquisition of a killer
disease called **"wasting disease"** or **"consumption,"** which eventually
killed twenty-three thousand people in just one day.

Led by the Holy Spirit and applying the Holy Bible as the acid
test to every vision, I undertook to understand the underlying philosophy surrounding *wasting disease.* My quest revealed that *wasting
disease* is synonymous with the HIV/AIDS scourge. Both have the same
characteristics.

What is wasting disease?

The Bible describes wasting disease as the kind of disease that consumes the flesh and deteriorates the body through rampant, uncontrollable fever and lack of nourishment, which cause the eyes to fail and life to ebb away. *This is exactly what AIDS does.*

The nature of wasting disease

- It was largely acquired via sexual immorality (character)
- It was also acquired via incision (custom)

Scripture tells us, "My people are destroyed for lack of knowledge [ignorance]."[2]

How wasting disease crept into the human race

Wasting disease, which is synonymous with AIDS, originated in Israel as a result of reckless sexual relationships between the Israelites and the Moabites in a place called Acacia Grove. The Moabites originated from incestuous relationships and formed a nation. According to God's instruction to the Israelites as His chosen people, they were to live separately from the Moabites. Since God had a plan for them as individuals and as a nation, He warned them not to mix with the inhabitants of other lands as they journeyed to the Promised Land. Specifically, they were not to engage in sexual relationships with them or serve their idols.

The Israelites, however, encamped in Acacia Grove in the Plains of Moab, and they did engage in sexual immorality with the people of Moab. God had warned that if they acted contrary to His commandments, they would suffer sudden terrors with wasting disease and with burning fevers that would cause their eyes to fail and life to recede. Because they did not obey God's command, a plague immediately broke out, and that plague was called **wasting disease.** In the words of

Numbers 25:1-2, "Now Israel remained in Acacia Grove and the people (the Israelites) began to commit harlotry with the women of Moab."[3]

Not only that, the people of Israel also accepted invitations from the Moabites to offer sacrifices and bow to their gods, in disobedience to God's command. "They invited the people to the sacrifices of their gods, and the people ate and bowed down to their gods. So Israel was joined to Baal of Peor, and the anger of the Lord was aroused against Israel."[4]

Since God had earlier warned them of the consequences of committing adultery and other acts of sexual immorality, as well as of the consequences of bowing down to idols or carved images, He punished their disobedience to His orders by allowing the wasting diseases already prevalent among the Moabites to come upon them. Scripture tells us,

> But if you do not obey Me, and do not observe all these commandments, and if you despise My statutes, or if your soul abhors My judgments, so that you do not perform all My commandments, but break My covenant, I also will do this you: I will even appoint terror over you, wasting disease and fever which shall consume the eyes and cause sorrow of heart.[5]

> Then, if you walk contrary to Me, and are not willing to obey Me, I will bring on you seven times more plagues, according to your sins.[6]

> Then the Lord will bring upon you and your descendants extraordinary plagues—great and prolonged plagues—and serious and prolonged sicknesses.[7]

A brief history of the Moabites

Moab is an ancient kingdom that was situated on a plateau to the east of the Dead Sea in what is now modern-day Jordan. Moab was the son of Lot's eldest daughter, born from the incest between father and daughter.

Lot had sexual relationships with his daughters, and they became pregnant as a result. The eldest daughter gave birth to a son and named him Moab, and he was the father of the Moabites. The younger daughter also gave birth to a son, and she named him Ben-ammi; he is the father of the people of Ammon. Lot and his daughter went against nature and committed the deepest dishonor to human nature. After this incestuous intercourse, Lot died in a cave.

How shameful Lot's family was! Moab and his mother were the first inhabitants of the land of Moab, and both the mother and her son are the progenitors of the Moabites. This brief history shows that the whole Moabite community was born out of most horrible incest. Therefore, the Moabites were already a sick community and were living with strange diseases, like wasting disease; that is why God said we should not go the way of immorality, for it has led others to the grave.

The consequences of disobedience

From the above Scriptural illustration, you can see that the Israelites did exactly what the Lord had commanded them *not* to do; they were enticed by the daughter of Moab both to whoredom and to idolatry. They provoked the Lord with their deeds, and a "plague" called "wasting disease" broke out among them, killing twenty-three thousand people in just one day. Before the plague could be stopped, it had wreaked havoc, killing up to twenty-four thousand people. *Plague is a disease that spreads rapidly through a population, killing a great many people.* A plague also can cause severe and lasting pain and other afflictions.

The Israelites were ignorant of two things about the Moabite community. First, during their idolatrous feasts, they engaged in gross sexual acts as a way of celebrating, and the majority already was living with a killer (wasting) disease, which is most often acquired via sexual immorality and did not show in their faces. Second, during this idolatrous feast, it was a common practice to make an incision, probably using the same blade for everyone, as a sign of submission to their god and to gain its protection.

This practice of incision was demonstrated when Prophet Elijah asked the prophets of Baal to prepare one bull, place it on wood, and then call out the name of their god. The Scriptures state that they called

Baal from morning until noon but received no sound or answer from a dead Baal.[8] They shouted loudly and cut themselves with knives and spears, according to their custom, until blood gushed out on them, but still there was no answer. Thus, the act of making incisions with a used blade became their custom and was another source of the spread of wasting disease within the Moabite community. In the twenty-first century, the act of incision has largely been replaced by body tattoos, which also result in the flow of blood. It would be good to remember that Scripture also says: "You are not to make gashes on your bodies for the dead or put tattoo marks on yourselves; I am the Lord."[9]

> ### *What is fashionable today could be*
> ### *a source of reproach tomorrow.*

Many regard body tattoos as fashionable, but any act that involves puncturing of the body to the point that blood comes out is like making a covenant to an unknown god, and this has implications for your life. What is fashionable today could be a source of reproach tomorrow. According to Deuteronomy 14:1-2:

> You are sons of the LORD your God; do not cut yourselves or make a bald spot on your head to an unknown god, for you are a holy people belonging to the LORD your God. The LORD has chosen you to be His special people out of all the people on the face of the earth.[10]

Knowledge of God shows that God does not destroy anyone; lack of knowledge, however, does destroy people.

Risky sex and sharing of sharp instruments are the two leading sources of HIV/AIDS.

According to Scripture, "Don't lust in your heart for her [an evil woman's], beauty or let her captivate you with her eyelashes."[11] The people completely forgot the deceptiveness of charm and the things that are hidden in beauty beyond the perception of ordinary eyes. No wonder the Scriptures also tell us not to follow the path of the immoral woman, for she has brought many down to death and her victims were strong men.[17] The Moabite women seduced the men with their beauty and charming eyelids. Some of these men followed the path of sexual immorality and acquired the killer disease. These acts of seduction marked the major starting point through which the Israelites acquired the killer disease. Today, sexual immorality constitutes the highest percentage of the incidence of HIV cases.

The Biblical wasting disease was not a contagious virus in the usual sense, because it was largely acquired from Moabite women through sexual acts, and no account showed that people got infected simply by sleeping or sitting together in the same camp or tent. Similarly, HIV is also not a contagious disease; it is mostly acquired via sexual immorality. Sleeping and sitting together do not spread HIV.

Wasting disease was so deadly in Biblical days that twenty-four thousand had died before someone's spirit was inspired by God to stand up and rebuke his brother when he came home with an immoral woman. Grieving and filled with fear, other people lent their support and eventually stopped the epidemic. They came together, worked together and stopped the epidemic. This is the starting point to defeat AIDS as John C. Maxwell said in *Think on These* Things, that "coming together is the beginning; working together produces victory."

Today, in a similar way, a pandemic called HIV/AIDS is killing thousands of people worldwide on a daily basis because of ignorance (lack of knowledge and understanding) and sexual immorality. Since the outbreak of this pandemic, more than twenty-five *million* people worldwide have died of AIDS. God has already said that no enchantment will hurt you and neither will any divination succeed against your family; and Christ has equally redeemed us from curses of the land; but the temptations of worldly interests and pleasures have brought back into society a *wasting disease* now known worldwide as HIV/AIDS.

This discovery was, to me, proof of the indisputable fact that, indeed, nothing is new under the sun. The ancient people were in close proximity to the Moabite city for nearly thirty-eight years. They were there long enough for any disease to manifest.

What went wrong in that century is what is going wrong in the twenty-first century: people suffer from ignorance and myopia in regard to the truth. They fell into sexual immorality. There are still 'Moabite' women and men in our society; they have migrated to every part of the world and are now living with HIV. What is more, they may try to seduce your friend, your brother, your sister, your children, and your spouse into sexual immorality because they lack knowledge and understanding of its consequences.

Be inspired to stand up and educate others and to correct every wrong behavior around you in order to fight the good fight against HIV/AIDS. This is how to come together and work together. Remember, God told us never to follow a crowd in wrongdoing. It is the responsibility of every person in every society, irrespective of age, location, and religion, to fight HIV/AIDS. The fight begins with you as a member of a family, which is the smallest unit in society. Writing this book is my own weapon to spread the knowledge and understanding of this epidemic, and I believe individual effort is what counts. I am standing with the Scriptures that say a threefold-cord is not quickly broken[12] and, without guidance, people fall. With many counselors, there is deliverance. I therefore humbly urge parents worldwide and all who are concerned to come together like a threefold cord and work together so that we can collectively, as one united family, change the face of AIDS. With this effort, we can exterminate AIDS. Everything is possible. Yes, it is.

CHAPTER TWO
THE ESSENCE OF BLOOD

It is really important to understand that life exists not in our flesh, but in our blood. The Scriptures say, "The life of a creature is in the blood."[1] Blood is an essential factor in determining well-being. Most people spend quality time taking care of their external bodies, not knowing that guarding the blood against destructive agents like HIV should be their main concern. Whatever affects the blood affects the body. The beauty of the body is in the blood, not in gold, jewelry, tattoos, and elegant clothes, which are merely decorative. If the blood is contaminated, the body is useless, no matter how strong or beautiful it is. Blood is life! HIV does not directly destroy the body; it destroys the blood, and whatever has the power to destroy the blood has equal power to destroy the body.

Your blood is your life.

We must do all we can to prevent the destruction of the blood by diseases like AIDS or wasting disease. The body must not be permitted to engage in sexual promiscuity, which directly exposes the blood to HIV. Disease poisons the blood. Like a rapid transit system, sexual immorality is a dedicated track that carries HIV rapidly and directly into the bloodstream. Therefore, sexual immorality is the cause of HIV rapid transmission (HRT). This definition fulfills and validates the fact that sexual immorality accounts for vast majority cases of HIV infection worldwide.

Sexual immorality is HIV rapid transmission (HRT).

Basic facts about white blood cells and HIV/AIDS

Human blood contains both red and white blood cells. These cells, particularly the white blood cells, are naturally positioned to defend and protect the human body against all kinds of diseases.

White blood cells are crucial to the normal function of the human immune system. Whenever a germ or infection enters the body, the white blood cells spontaneously move toward the scene and attack the invader by producing protective antibodies that are capable of subduing it and preventing the body from being destroyed.

It is important at this point to acquaint you with the hostile relationship between white blood cells and HIV. When HIV invades the body, it attacks the white blood cells in human blood, thereby destroying the body's defense system making it susceptible to deadly infections.

When the Human Immunodeficiency Virus is present in the body, it resides in the body fluids, especially in white blood cells, and HIV has devices that it uses to attack the white blood cells, making them less effective.

White Blood Cell

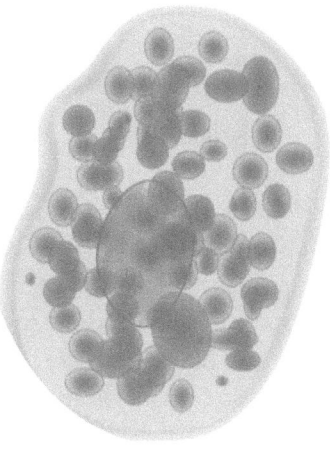

What is HIV?

HIV stands for Human Immunodeficiency Virus. It enters human blood through sexual intercourse, the shared use of sharp objects, or through blood transfusion. A virus is a small germ (smaller than a bacterium) that causes an infectious disease. The human immunodeficiency virus specifically seeks to destroy the life-giving blood. After the HIV virus has attacked and weakened the body, it develops into AIDS, which has power to ravage and finally kill the human body. The conflict of interest between this invader and the defending white blood cells continues for as long as one is able to overpower the other. And so, the battle is waged.

White blood cells defend the body and attack diseases that threaten us.

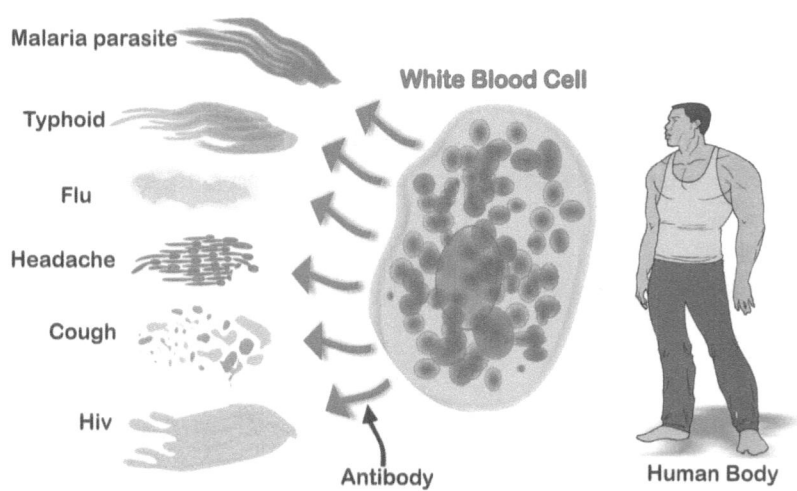

The picture above depicts a scenario in which the body is under serious attack by malaria parasite, typhoid, headache, flu, cough, and HIV, which is the deadliest of them all. Their first priority is to attack the blood; as soon as the white blood cells foresee the attack, on their own volition, they build a fence or wall of antibodies around the body to defend it, thereby blocking out the invader. To use a war analogy, the antibodies are fired like weapons to subdue the enemy. In football, this would be called the defensive strategy. Penetrating this defense is difficult for some diseases. HIV, however, attaches itself to the blood to drain off energy and life by vigorously feeding on the nutrients the blood uses for growth, as depicted in the diagram below.

HIV feeding on the Nutrients
that the Blood Uses for Body Growth

White Blood Cell

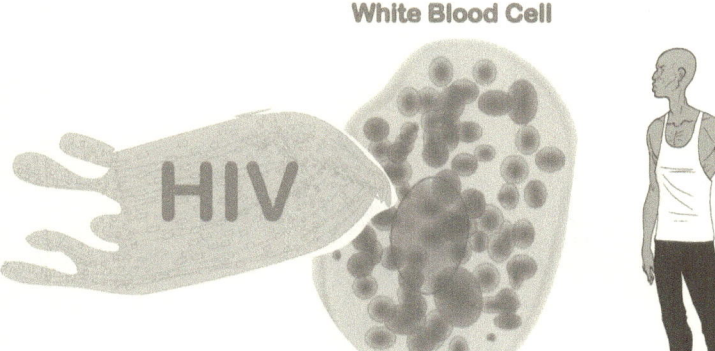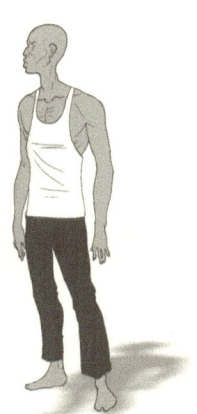

Human Body

1. The white blood cell defends the body and attacks parasites. All the other diseases that attack the body are contained by the antibodies that the white blood cells produce. Only HIV remains adamant, because it is a stronger virus. This development allows HIV to penetrate the blood and multiply by feeding on the nutrients in the blood until it multiplies and gains enough power to destroy the body). HIV depends on the nutrients in the blood to multiply, and as it multiplies, the body weakens.

At this juncture, there are certain things you need to understand.

- The attack on the blood by HIV signifies the beginning of a big battle for supremacy, and this can continue for as long as the white blood cells are still very active.

- HIV seems to understand the rules of war; it uses tactics like eating up the energy nutrients provided by the cells for growth and reproduction. Gradually, this weakens and breaks down the white blood cells, reducing their effectiveness in fighting against diseases and infections.

- Based on these excellent tactics by the HIV virus, we can therefore conclude that the HIV virus is stronger than the white blood cells.

2. Once the HIV virus has rendered the white blood cells less effective in protecting the body system and fighting diseases, the diseases can enter and kill the victim.

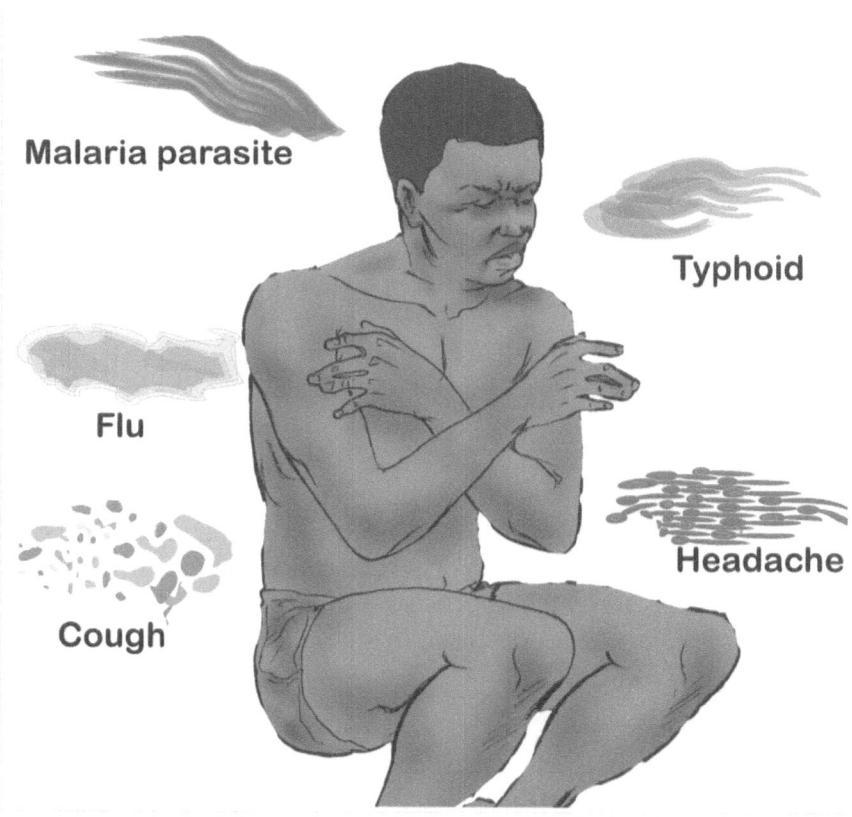

At the stage illustrated above, the body is extremely helpless, the blood is contaminated, and the body is directly exposed to the HIV virus and other various opportunistic infections. The more the HIV virus multiplies, the more it weakens the immune system and leaves the person vulnerable to illnesses ranging from pneumonia to cancer.

The obvious conclusion is that it is better to avoid HIV rather than to acquire it and manage it. Being infected with HIV provides the gateway for other diseases.

NOTE: Due to HIV, diseases such as the malaria parasite can easily enter the body system, and malaria kills faster than HIV/AIDS. Malaria has a cure, but HIV/AIDS is yet to have a cure. Consult medical personnel for every kind of treatment. Do not subject yourself to self-medication; go for a medical checkup.

What is AIDS?

AIDS stands for "Acquired Immunodeficiency Syndrome." It is a disease by which the flesh is consumed and the whole body is dried up by rampant fever as a result of lack of nourishment. This disease occurs when HIV virus cling to the human blood for a long time, extracting nutrients for its own advantage and gaining more energy every day. When it makes the body weak enough, HIV develops into the more deadly and life-destroying disease now widely called **AIDS**. The manifestation at this stage is a collection of sicknesses combined with bodily degeneration that result when the immune system can no longer effectively defend and protect the body. These sicknesses include frequent fever, skin rashes, cough, loss of weight, and diarrhea. All these illnesses are called opportunistic infections because they take advantage of a weakened immune system. This situation would not have occurred if HIV had not made the white blood cells less effective.

As I stated previously, the Biblical name for AIDS is *wasting disease.*

How HIV develops into AIDS

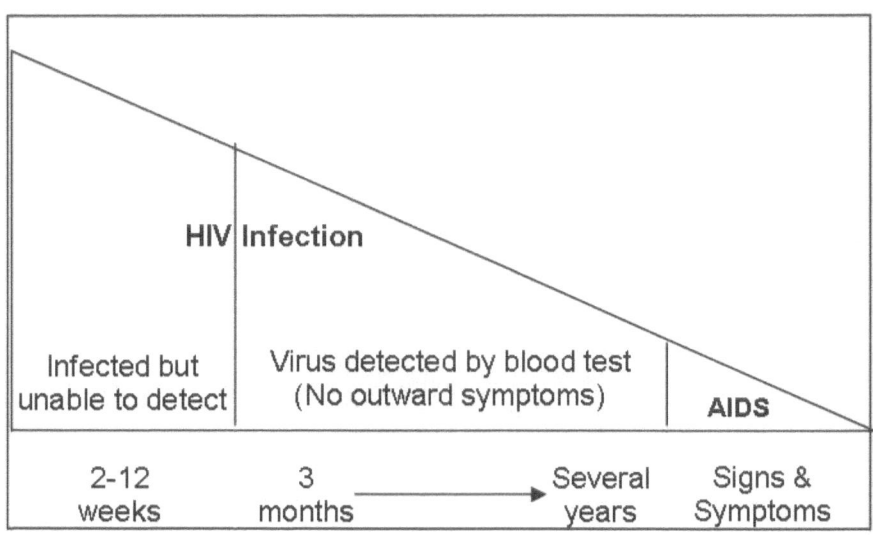

- From 2-12 weeks of being infected with HIV is what is called the Window Period. During this time, the virus cannot be detected with the usual blood-screening techniques, however the virus may be present, and it can be transmitted. This period is very dangerous because it can give a false indication of a person's HIV status. Consequently, any blood test should be repeated after approximately three months. The outcome of this new test will be the starting point for determining further action.

- From 3 months to several years after infection, the virus can only be detected by blood-screening techniques. During this period, an infected person will look very beautiful, handsome, strong, elegant, robust, and healthy, because *HIV DOES NOT SHOW IN SOMEONE'S FACE.* HIV is a deceptive and misleading disease since how a person looks does not reflect his or her HIV status. Only a blood-screening technique or test will give an accurate negative or positive result. During this second stage of the disease, antiretroviral drugs can be used to energize the white blood cells in order to delay the progression of HIV into AIDS.

Do you now understand that millions of people are walking around with the HIV virus? They could be your best friends, neighbors, business partners, students, teachers, or managers. Having HIV/AIDS is hidden, a secret the victims will not discuss with you for fear of discrimination, isolation, and neglect. HIV does not show in someone's face. We all need knowledge and understanding to protect ourselves from being infected.

3. After stages 1 and 2, HIV develops into the more deadly virus AIDS, which presents several symptoms and body degeneration. At stage 3 of this disease, there will be rigorous manifestation of other diseases, along with body degeneration.

Can any HIV-positive person avoid full-blown AIDS?

Yes, it is possible if the HIV virus is detected by a blood test early enough, as in stage 2. In that case, medical personnel can help manage the virus properly. When it is allowed to develop into full-blown AIDS, it becomes fatal and is an open secret.

Ignorance is a disease deadlier than AIDS. Our first assignment is to fight ignorance with knowledge and understanding. If we can defeat ignorance, then we have defeated AIDS.

Global estimates for adults and children living with HIV Infection worldwide

The AIDS outbreak is one of the greatest threats facing our world today. No country is in any way safe, irrespective of economic power or life expectancy. HIV/AIDS cases have been reported in almost every nook and cranny of the world.

The joint United Nations Program on HIV/AIDS (UNAIDS) statistically puts the number of people living with HIV as over 40 million people worldwide as of the end of 2005, 39.5 million in 2006, and 33.2 million in 2007, of which the majority are ignorant of their HIV status and may be spreading the virus to others. From 2005 to 2007, progress has been made, but the number is still much too high, and much must be done to defeat HIV.

2007 AIDS Epidemic Update
GLOBAL OVERVIEW[3]

Number of people living with HIV in 2007

Total 33.2 million (30.6 - 36.1 million)

Adults – 30.8 million (28.2 - 33.6 million)

Women – 15.4 million (13.9 - 16.6 million)

Children under 15 years – 2.5 million (2.2 – 2.6 million)

People newly infected with HIV in 2007

Total 2.5 million (1.8 - 4.1 million)

Adults -- 2.1 million (1.4 - 3.6 million)

Children under 15 years – 420,000 (350,000 - 540,000)

AIDS deaths in 2007

Total 2.1 million (1.9 – 2.4 million)

Adults – 1.7 million (1.6 – 2.1 million)

Children under 15 years – 330,000 (310,000 – 380,000)

The ranges around the estimates in this table define the boundaries around the actual numbers, based on the best available information. The estimated average number of persons living with HIV worldwide in 2007 was 33.2 million, a reduction of 16 percent compared with the estimated average 39.5 million published in 2006.

Ever since this outbreak began, it has been documented that more than 25 million people have died from AIDS worldwide, more than from malaria and tuberculosis. It is the most deadly infectious disease among adults and is the fourth leading cause of death worldwide. Fifteen million children have been orphaned by AIDS (www.unaids. org). This figure is high, and today it is on the rise. Two and a half million people became infected in 2007 alone, and more people are getting infected every day, simply because they lack understanding. *What about you?*

How does one acquire HIV/AIDS?

HIV is not a contagious disease; hence, it cannot be passed by merely sitting next to or hugging an infected person. It is chiefly spread from one immoral person to another immoral person. However, there are several other ways through which someone can, through lack of knowledge, acquire the disease: HIV is found in human body fluids, such as blood, semen, breast milk, and fluid from a woman's vagina. However, specific actions must be taken to acquire HIV from these body fluids.

A disease can either be "contagious," meaning that it is communicable, or "acquired," meaning that it is obtained only through certain actions. HIV/AIDS can be acquired through the following actions:

1. **Reckless sex (destructive sex):** This involves sexual relations between two people who are not yet married (premarital sex) or married people who engage in sexual relationships outside the marital bond. Semen and vaginal fluids carry higher amounts of the HIV virus than any other body fluids. Having sex with an HIV-infected person, whether it is oral, vaginal, or anal sex, will expose you to the highest risk of HIV infection. It was through reckless sexual relationships that people in Biblical times acquired wasting disease, and they died.

Indulgence in reckless sex is the most dangerous enemy to your life. Reckless sex gives satisfaction to your body, but it destroys your soul. Which is more important to you? Your soul is the energy of your destiny. When your soul is destroyed, your future is destroyed. We have been told to wear condoms to prevent sexual disease, but there are no protective materials that will prevent the soul from destruction. Over eighty percent of people living with HIV/AIDS got infected through reckless sex. Sex is heartwarming and uncontrollably inspiring to the human body, but it also has the power to wreck the greatest dream and dreamer. This is why the Scripture says, "Stolen water is sweet, and bread eaten in secret is pleasant, but the consequence is the mark of everlasting destruction."[4]

2. **Anal and oral-genital sex:** Anal sex is sex through the anus, while oral-genital sex involves the mouth and the sex organs. Men and women who practice oral-genital sex are at risk for HIV infection, and even more so when it is engaged in with many sex partners or when ejaculation occurs in the mouth. This risk gets even higher when either partner has abrasions, cuts, or sores, such as canker or other sores caused by sexually transmitted diseases (STD) or recent tooth-brushing, because these also allow the virus to enter the bloodstream. Anal sex (whether male-female, male-male, or female–female) puts you at high risk of contracting HIV because the lining of the anus and the rectum is extremely thin and is filled with small blood

vessels that can easily break during intercourse, permitting HIV virus to enter.

3. **Sharing of used and unsterilized sharp objects:** If you share needles, syringes, razor blades, scissors, knives, barber clippers, and other sharp objects with an HIV-infected person, you will expose yourself to a very high risk of contracting the virus.

When any razor, knife, or sharp object mistakenly cuts through the skin and touches the blood of an infected person, the object becomes infected with the virus; any re-use by another person will spread the disease to him or her, especially when the instrument has not been properly sterilized. Studies have confirmed that HIV is spread at an alarming rate through this practice.

Consider the following:

• **Shaving and barbering with unsterilized blades**

Good grooming makes you more respectable and shows you to be worthy of responsibility, but shaving and barbering with unsterilized objects can put you at risk of HIV infection.

• **Cutting your nails with unsterilized blades**

Our nails should be trimmed, but borrowing nail clippers or getting your nails cut in a public shop and with unsterilized blades can subject people to HIV. Be careful how you cut your nails. It is safer to buy your own manicure or pedicure kit. Always remember that negligence can be costly.

• **Body tattooing**

You may consider body tattooing, which I call modern incision, fashionable, but it is a common way of acquiring HIV when done in public shops or at home with an unsterilized instrument. Remember, worldly interests and pleasures have a price tag.

Furthermore, any act in which you cut your body, causing blood to ooze or flow, symbolically shows that you are making a covenant to an unknown god, and this has implications for your life. *Remember, what is fashionable today could be a source of reproach tomorrow.*

- **Traditions that pave the way for acquiring HIV**

Circumcision, incisions, and tribal marks are part of some traditions or customs, but parents must be careful not to use unsterilized blades. Tribal marks were fashionable in earlier times, but today nobody wants to be identified with them because they lead to acquiring HIV. Constitutionally, tribal marks should be banned.

HIV can survive in used syringes for a long time, and this necessitates that hospitals and social health workers, as well as parents who perform circumcisions, incisions, and body tattooing, should be well educated against re-use of unsterilized instruments, such as syringes, blades, and needles. All of these are good harbors for HIV. Such education is essential to avoiding the possibility that someone's negligence or action will destroy another person's life, especially the life of an infant, who has no control over such activities.

4. **Unscreened blood transfusion:** You can get infected when HIV-infected blood mixes with your blood. This can happen via a blood transfusion. Before you accept a blood transfusion, ask if the blood has been properly screened and, if possible, check the label to ascertain this or request that the doctor sign a written statement as to the credibility of the blood's status. It is your right to know so that someone's negligence will not cost you your life.

5. **From mother to baby:** An HIV-positive woman can pass the virus on to her baby. The baby becomes infected while in the mother's womb, during delivery, or during breastfeeding. This is why it is most advisable that a mother be tested so that she does not unintentionally pass the virus on to her baby.

Medical science has devised a means to prevent the infant from getting infected, which means that an HIV-positive mother can give birth to an HIV-negative infant, but this is based strictly on following medical practices and advice. Save the life of your child by seeking medical help.

Wrong notions about acquiring HIV

Some people wrongly believe that HIV can be transmitted by sitting beside an HIV-infected person or by touching, hugging, kissing, shaking hands, playing, sleeping, or eating with an HIV-infected person. All these beliefs are quite mistaken. They are myths and do not have an iota of truth.

You cannot acquire HIV from:

- **Hugging:** You cannot acquire HIV by hugging an infected person, because HIV is not a contagious disease. However, you must be careful not to engage in hugging that can lead to immoral behavior. Hugging is a sign of love, not sex.

- **Shaking hands:** You cannot acquire HIV by shaking hands with an infected person, because HIV is not a contagious disease. A handshake is a greeting or an expression of pleasantries. It engenders friendship. HIV is a virus that lives in human blood and not on the hands.

- **Eating together:** Eating with an HIV-infected person will not put you at risk, and you will not acquire HIV by eating from the same plate as an infected person. HIV does not live on any external part of the body; it lives in the blood and in the internal regions of the human body. Eating together is a sign of love and togetherness.

- **Sharing a comb:** You cannot acquire HIV from an infected person from sharing a comb or brush, because HIV is not a contagious disease, but do not share a comb that has a sharp enough edge to cause bleeding of the scalp.

- **Sitting close:** Sitting close to an infected person does not spread HIV. A countless number of situations require us to sit next to others, such as on the bus or in various social assemblies. Doing so will not put you at risk.

- **Insect bites:** You cannot acquire HIV from insect bites. Mosquitoes, bedbugs, and the like can only spread malaria, which, unlike AIDS, is easily transmissible from one person to another. Therefore, being in the same neighborhood with an HIV-infected person will not put you at risk.

- **Toilets:** Toilets do not spread HIV, because HIV is not a contagious disease. Nevertheless, it is always a good idea to wash your hands with soap and water afterwards.

Symptoms of AIDS

As explained earlier, AIDS manifests as a myriad of sicknesses, and these cause a further breakdown of the body's immune system. These sicknesses arise after HIV has weakened the body. HIV that has been in the body for a long time without being medically treated will eventually turn into full-blown AIDS.

People living with AIDS get sicknesses such as:

- **Tuberculosis:** Having tuberculosis could be a sign of AIDS, but a medical test is needed to ascertain this. Tuberculosis, usually called TB, is a serious disease which usually attacks the lungs but can also affect other parts of the body. TB is an infectious disease. A persistent, troublesome cough needs urgent medical attention to ascertain its cause.

- **Diarrhea:** In this illness, there is frequent emptying of waste matter from the bowels in liquid form. Diarrhea leads to quick weight loss. Persistent and unexplained diarrhea, the source of which cannot be established, could be a sign of AIDS.

- **Fever:** This is a condition in which a person has a higher-than-normal temperature that often brings on chills. Medical tests may indicate any of the following: glandular fever, hay fever, malaria fever, rheumatic fever, scarlet fever, or yellow fever. A fever that resists treatment and persists for a long time could be a sign of AIDS.

- **Flu:** Flu is a disease that can be passed from one person to another. It comes on in the form of a very serious cold that causes fever, pain, and body aches. If flu persists for an unusually long time and defies medical treatment, it might be a symptom of AIDS.

- **Skin rashes:** Rashes are red spots on the skin. Usually, they are caused by an illness or a reaction to some food, drug, cloth, heat, or anything else that comes in contact with the skin.

Manifestation of red spots all over the body with significant and unexplained weight loss could be a sign of AIDS.

It should be noted that there are other symptoms of AIDS. However, you cannot rely on symptoms to conclude that someone who is suffering from any of the above-mentioned illnesses is an AIDS-infected person. Only medical tests can establish the presence of HIV in the human body. Only a medical diagnosis can determine whether an illness is a sign of AIDS.

CHAPTER THREE
Means to Identify the AIDS Virus

The most recognized means to identify the HIV virus is through a special blood test known as the HIV/AIDS test, which can establish whether the HIV virus is present in the blood stream. When a person is infected with HIV, his or her immune system tries to fight the virus by creating antibodies. Antibodies are one of the body's tools for fighting infection. An HIV test looks for the presence of HIV antibodies. If antibodies to HIV are present, the person is HIV-infected.

Most hospitals and medical laboratories are well equipped to carry out HIV tests. The HIV test should be analyzed by a medical laboratory and not by a pharmacy outlet. There should always be a counselor available to explain all you need to know about the HIV test.

Can you tell who has HIV/AIDS?

You absolutely *cannot* tell by looking whether someone is HIV-positive. Only a medical test can determine who is HIV-positive. Every time I come across a military person or a policeman, I can easily identify him or her by the uniform. I also can often identify a corporate executive or a medical doctor by what he or she is wearing, but when I come across a beautiful woman or a handsome man in nice clothes, I remember this fact: *HIV DOES NOT SHOW ON A PERSON'S FACE.* You cannot tell merely by looking at a person's presentation whether he or she has HIV. The Moabite women were described as extremely beautiful, yet they were living with wasting disease.

An HIV test is the only way to verify a person's HIV status. *AIDS is quite common and AIDS presently has no cure! Beauty and attire can be deceptive. Things may be hidden in beauty that ordinary eyes cannot see, and most of these things are life-destroyers. Therefore, it is always necessary to know the HIV status of a person with whom you intend to have a romantic relationship.*

Is an HIV test a necessity?

There are many beautiful people in the world today who are living with HIV, and as I have emphasized, no one can judge any human being according to appearances. A blood test is necessary to determine HIV status.

- Testing is necessary in order to ascertain your own HIV/AIDS status.

- Testing is necessary in order to diagnose the sickness in a timely manner, before it gets out of control. An early diagnosis will help people who are HIV-positive to live a normal life and a longer life.

- A test allows newly infected people to register for clinical care. Many people are living with the HIV virus without receiving any medical care, just because they do not know they have the disease. Testing will help people living with the HIV virus to start receiving anti-retroviral drugs that can help them live a healthier, happier, and longer life.

- Testing will make an infected person conscious of his status so that he does not ignorantly spread the disease to others, including family members.

- Testing is necessary for pregnant women. Infected mothers can bottle-feed instead of breastfeed to avoid spreading the disease to their babies through breast milk.

- Many beautiful women and handsome men are living with HIV these days. Young couples are advised to undergo HIV testing to determine their status before they enter into any serious relationship.

- Testing enables patients to know in advance the condition of the blood that may be given to them. If need be, patients must insist on HIV-screened blood before receiving any blood. Medical experts also have a responsibility to ensure that all blood is well screened before giving transfusions. It is cruel and unprofessional to transfuse untested blood to patients.

- Testing gives medical experts information on the number of people infected with HIV and their general location. It helps them to monitor the progress of the epidemic. No medical professional will ever reveal or make public your medical record to anyone.

- Last, testing helps medical service personnel to determine the impact of their prevention efforts aimed at reducing the epidemic.

Why people run away from the HIV test

An HIV/AIDS test is a must before marriage, before deciding to have a baby, and especially if you think you have engaged in reckless sex or other such risky behavior.

People are afraid of the results. If you have been exposed to reckless sex, avoiding the reality of testing to confirm your HIV/AIDS status can be dangerous. You can ignorantly infect your family members, friends, colleagues, and loved ones.

- Some people may have been involved in risky things, like having sex with prostitutes or with many partners or sharing needles. Such people may be uncomfortable discussing HIV because they are not proud of their activities.

- Stigmatization associated with HIV has created fear in the hearts of many people, who believe that offering to take a test is an indication of involvement in risky behaviors. This is not the case. Taking an HIV/AIDS test means that you are wise enough to save your life as well as protect others.

It does not matter what your feelings are. Feeling bad about your recent activities will create fear of going for an HIV test, but you need to realize that testing will make you aware of your HIV status, and that has the potential to make you avoid any further risky behavior. Not only that, but if you discover that you have the disease, it will encourage you to urgently seek medical assistance so that you can have access to drugs that will make the virus inactive for as long as possible.

HIV test results

HIV test results can identify and validate the presence of antibodies in the blood as early as thirteen weeks after infection, although the body may take up to six months to make a measurable amount of antibodies. The average time needed to build up measurable antibodies is twenty-five days. Your HIV test result will be either positive or negative.

- A **positive** result means that you are already infected with the HIV virus. At this stage, it is important to respond positively and follow available professional advice. Remember, *a positive result is not a death sentence.* What is required is the ability to choose hope over fear, because fear repels miracles. It takes between six months and several years for HIV to fully manifest into AIDS. Drug treatments that can further delay the development of HIV into AIDS are available.

Fear repels miracles.

- A **negative** result indicates that you are not infected with HIV. Congratulations on this result, but that does not make you better than people who are positive. This is why society must accord people who are positive respect, care, and unconditional love, without discrimination. If you test negative, it is medically advisable that you be retested every six months, because it can take up to six months for the immune system to produce enough antibodies to show up on the test. People in this category should be careful not to think that being HIV-negative is a passport to engage in any indecent behavior.

Anyone who has received an HIV test should seek counseling before and after the test in order to understand the results and discuss prevention methods and drug treatment options.

Privacy and testing

It is important for anyone having an HIV test to understand the confidentiality policies of the testing center. The only people with access to your test results are medical personnel and you. Medical personnel have been trained not to disclose any secrets relating to the health condition of their patients. In this regard, anything less than this complete confidentiality is professional misconduct and is a criminal offense that is punishable by law.

CHAPTER FOUR
FORMULA TO PREVENT HIV INFECTION

The most excellent and most guaranteed means to prevent or defeat HIV/AIDS in our world today is to imbibe the spoken words of Almighty God and establish the standards of God in our hearts as our daily principles.

The Scriptures say,

It [This teaching of God] will keep you from the immoral woman,

from the smooth tongue of an adulterous woman.

Don't lust for her beauty.

Don't let her coyness seduce you.

For a prostitute will bring you to poverty,

and sleeping with another man's wife may cost you your very life.

Can a man scoop fire into his lap and not be burned?

Can that same man walk on hot coals and not blister his feet?

So it is with the man who sleeps with another man's wife.

He who embraces her will not go unpunished.[1]

For by means of a harlot a man is reduced to a crust of bread; and an adulteress will prey upon his precious life[2]

The words quoted above are what I consider the Almighty's formula to save our souls, which are very precious to God. In regard to HIV, anyone who engages in sexual immorality is at high risk for contracting the disease, which has the power to destroy the soul. Remember, the energy of your destiny is your soul. Our duty is to be guided by this moral principle so that we can protect our souls. Engaging in protective sex cannot in any way protect our souls.

And so, the formula for saving our souls includes:

- Total abstinence from sex is your best option for avoiding HIV. It is the only option that is 100 percent risk-free

- If you are married, remaining faithful to your spouse is crucial for avoiding HIV/AIDS. Infidelity is a silent destroyer of marriage and destiny.

> *Infidelity is a silent destroyer of marriage and your God-given destiny.*

Remember, infidelity will put not only you but also your entire family at great risk of acquiring HIV/AIDS. Think about this: Would you rather destroy your destiny or protect it? The choice is completely yours, and your choices define your lot. How would you feel if you caught your wife or husband cheating on you before your very eyes? I do not know what your answer is, but hear what God tells us about the unfaithful person: "He [She] will be wounded and disgraced. His [Her] shame will never be erased."[3] I command the spirit of infidelity to come out of you and never go back again.

- The world has told us that protected sex will *minimize* the risk of getting infected, NOT *maximize* it. Any measure that minimizes but does not maximize the risk of HIV infection can also be regarded as one that supports reckless behavior. Protective measures are not 100 percent risk-free. For instance, protective sex cannot guarantee safety, because a condom can tear, so if you rely on it in cases where the HIV status of your sexual partner is not known, you put yourself at a greater risk. Sexual immorality is also a soul-sinker, because there are no condoms to protect your soul.

There are no condoms to protect your soul

Other means to prevent HIV are:

- Do not share instruments such as razor blades, needles, and syringes. If sharing is a must, then insist on using sterilized instruments.

- If you have any cut or wound on your body, please cover it well with a waterproof bandage or a piece of clean cloth.

- Before marriage, both partners must undergo an HIV/AIDS test. Do not have sex until you are legally married and then be faithful to your partner.

- Women with HIV should seek advice before getting pregnant because they can pass on HIV to their babies. Medical assistance can go a long way to assist them in preventing possible harm to their unborn babies.

- Breast milk is the best food for a newborn baby. An infant deserves the natural milk from its mother's breast, which protects the baby against many infant killer diseases. However, the possibility of an HIV-positive mother transmitting the virus to her baby through breastfeeding is extremely high. Nursing mothers who are HIV-positive should not breastfeed their babies; they should seek alternative feeding methods. Information on alternative feeding methods for babies is available upon request in hospitals and health care centers.

Examine the options below and make a better choice today.

Abstinence is 100 percent risk-free. It is a life-saving decision. It is a life of moral excellence. Abstaining from sex is possible because, as the Scripture says, "Everything is possible."

Reckless Sex is zero percent risk-free. Even one night of reckless sex can bring misfortune and great disaster. Reckless sex will clothe your destiny in rags.

41

Infidelity is a burning candle that can turn your destiny into ashes.

Sharing used sharp objects, as, for example, when you get a shave, a manicure, or a pedicure in a shop, is another practice that shows lack of understanding and wisdom when it comes to the issue of HIV/AIDS and its consequent destruction.

Sex before marriage could ruin your destiny.

Sex before marriage (pre-marital sex) is dangerous. When rain starts falling early in the morning and continues until late in the night, people with understanding carry an umbrella to prevent getting soaked. Pre-marital sex can soak your future with regrets and agonies, and if care is not taken, you might live to regret it for the rest of your life. It does not matter whether you have already had sex; you can start abstaining from sex from now on. Abstaining from sex before marriage is absolutely possible, because "everything is possible."

The above are the available options to safeguard your destiny. I am challenging you to make the right decisions. *YOUR CHOICE IS WHO YOU ARE.* Decide where you belong on the axis, for every destination begins with a decision. If you desire to achieve greatness in life, **then learn to do it right by living right.** You need to understand that living right comes with a price tag, but your decision to pay the price now will deliver a better destiny to you later. Living right might come with pain, as well, but it is better to experience the pain of self-discipline now than to bear the burden of regret later. Discipline is the link between your desire and your success.

What exactly is the price you must pay to live correctly?

The price you must pay is the self-discipline to abstain from sex before entering into a safe marriage. If you can delay gratification and practice complete **abstinence**, you are on the right course. Do not pay attention to what the environment is saying or what your friends are doing. You can make a difference; do not follow the crowd to do evil. Decide today to deny your body the worldly pleasure it derives from unholy sex. This decision might be a hard-hitting one, but it is also a life-saving decision. If you can stand by it, you have secured your destiny, *which is greatness.*

Your choice is who you are. Your destiny is too precious, and nothing should stop you in life, not even a relationship that demands sex as a precondition for marriage. Sex before marriage is a cancer on your rightful destiny, and abstaining from sex before marriage is absolutely possible because "everything is possible."

Can HIV be cured?

There have been several attempts to find a cure for HIV/AIDS. Medical scientists have intensified their efforts towards producing an antidote for HIV/AIDS, exploring all possible means within their reach. Their efforts have yielded success in the area of producing antiretroviral drugs to treat HIV infection but, at present, there are no acceptable drugs for the cure of HIV. Some of these drugs are designed to prevent HIV itself from reproducing and destroying the body's immune system.

For proper treatment, please seek the advice of medical personnel. Abiding by the axiom, "Prevention is better than a cure," this book can serve as a critical resource for knowledge and understanding of HIV/AIDS. Knowledge and understanding are crucial for avoiding and preventing this epidemic. AIDS presently has no scientific cure, but embracing and practicing God's principles can exterminate AIDS.

Recently, a woman shared her testimony as to how the anointing of God destroyed the yoke of this scourge and healed her. As she spoke, she was holding her medical report as proof that she is now testing negative for HIV. I believe in my heart that her testimony was the fulfillment of the Scripture that says, "In that day the LORD will end the bondage of his people. He will break the yoke of slavery and lift it from their shoulders."[4],--meaning that to him who believes in God "everything is possible."

As you adhere to medical instruction and take your drugs, you can equally put your trust in God for your healing, and I am sure the anointing of God will destroy the yoke of every sickness in your life. Having heard this awesome testimony, God is on the throne of grace, dispensing His anointing, and very soon the world will acquire the wisdom to produce the Almighty's formula, which will lead to the permanent cure for HIV, in the name of Jesus.

This is prophetic, but I want you all to agree in the unity of hearts that "God has spoken, and who can change His plans? When His hand moves, who can stop him?"[5] Yes, no one can stop the Almighty's formula, which will produce healing drugs for over 30 million people who are living with HIV worldwide, because only God can solve a problem that defies human solution. I believe in my heart that we should throw over earthly wisdom and look up to heaven for the cure, because the cure might not be as complex as we thought. What is humanly impossible is possible with God. Impossibility is merely ignorance. God's wisdom can do all things. "Everything is possible."

Impossibility is just ignorance of possibility.

Looking healthy with HIV/AIDS

Since a permanent cure has not been formulated for AIDS, the best way any positive person can look healthy is to be under treatment and try to eat good, nutritious food. Remember, God is the greatest healer; putting your faith in Him will compel the universe to deliver your healing. Talk to your health care provider regularly, just to stay informed and keep your viral load as low as possible. God bless you.

Practical ways to live successfully when you are HIV/AIDS-positive

- Keep your body active by singing and dancing, which are signs of positive living. These will energize you and increase your hope.

- By all means, avoid alcoholic drinks and smoking. These two things can create depression, and depression can quicken HIV into AIDS.

- Keep your body clean, tidy, and healthy by practicing good hygiene.

- Sleeping refreshes the brain. HIV-positive people should get maximum rest, as this will help them to keep fit.

- Getting good medical treatment will help delay the progression of HIV into AIDS.

- The body needs nutritious food to function effectively. An HIV-positive person should eat a healthy diet. According to Scripture, "I tell you, you can pray for anything, and if you believe that you've received it, it will be yours."[6] If you desire a miracle, this is how it works: Place your faith in Christ and believe that, by His grace, you will be healed. Faith brings healing, while fear repels the miraculous. Remain under medical treatment, and your miracle will land soon.

Caring for children who have HIV/AIDS

Children with HIV/AIDS need affection. Parents, friends, relatives, governments, NGOs, religious groups, and society at large should give them maximum love. A child with HIV/AIDS has every right to a quality education and good food. Parents must:

- Feed children properly, as this will help them stay healthy and keep fit.

- Make sure they get maximum treatment for opportunistic infections as early as possible.

- Make sure they are well immunized against all diseases.

- Show them deep and genuine love and allow them to play with others. The Bible tells us that, through love, we should serve one another.

How your community can help People Living with HIV/ AIDS (PLWHA)

- Avoid discrimination and stigmatization of PLWHA.
- Within your own small capacity, provide care and support to PLWHA.
- Always respect the rights of PLWHA.
- Show PLWHA maximum love, as this will strengthen them and make them feel more comfortable about relating with others.
- Pay attention to the needs of PLWHA.

- Donate whatever small amount you can to support PLWHA. As the opportunity presents itself, please be good to all, especially to those who are critically in need of your help. *"Do not withhold good from those to whom it is due when it is in the power of your hand to do so."* [7]
- Pray for PLWHA. As the Scripture says, "The prayer of faith will save the sick and the Lord will raise him up. And if he has committed sins, he will be forgiven. Confess your trespasses one to another, and pray one for another, that you may be healed."[7]

The rights of People Living with HIV/AIDS

At this juncture, we need to understand that HIV/AIDS is a public health problem. It is not inherited and could happen to anyone. In this regard, people living with HIV/AIDS have the same fundamental human rights as every other person. Some of the internationally accepted human rights include:

- The right to life

- The right to health care
- The right to shelter
- The right to education
- The right to dignity
- The right to gender equality
- The right to employment
- The right to freedom of speech and expression
- The right to freedom of religion
- The right to vote and to be voted for
- The right to the basic amenities of life
- The right to love and to be loved

People living with HIV/AIDS are God's creatures, the same as all other individuals in the world. They deserve our sincere love and our respect. Let us accord them the regard and love that can increase self-esteem.

CHAPTER FIVE
SEX

Sex is a special gift to humanity. Sex is socially acceptable and fulfilling, but only in the context of marriage. It can be destructive outside a marital relationship. Marriage is a legal, documented, and mutual agreement between a man and a woman to live together as one. In this regard, sex is the channel through which the blessing of procreation takes place, fulfilling the Scripture that says, ". . . be fruitful, multiply, and replenish the earth, and subdue it . . ."[1] It can therefore be said that, in marriage, sex is a most beautiful and gratifying act, while outside of marriage, sex is pointless, needless, unjustifiable, and destructive to the soul.

Before marriage, partners are advised to take an HIV test to ascertain their status. After that, having sex in marriage becomes quite safe, provided both partners remain faithful to each other. If both partners remain faithful and do not engage in other risky practices that can transmit HIV, as detailed earlier in the book, sex can be regarded as safe because it is absolutely permitted and does not transmit HIV/AIDS or any other sexually transmitted disease.

ENJOYABLE SEX	DESTRUCTIVE SEX
Sex in the context of marriage	Premarital sex
	Same-sex partners (Gays/Lesbians)
	Incest and sexual assault

Wholesome sex

By wholesome sex, I mean sex in the context of marriage. It is socially acceptable, decent, desirable, and to be encouraged. The results of such sex are:

- It will create a strong bond between a husband and wife.
- It will lead to procreation, to having good children.
- It is the pride of every family.
- It is fully sanctified.
- It is a dream come true.
- It is an appreciation of love between a husband and wife.
- It will enrich the partners' souls.
- It is not impure.
- It is a beautiful thing.
- It was created and designed by God.

Destructive sex

Destructive sex is any sex that takes place outside of marriage, such as sex before marriage or sex between homosexuals. It is destructive and unacceptable because it is immoral. It is a dream killer, and its consequences are always enormous, unbearable, unimaginable, and unspeakable. The consequences are:

- It creates reproach between irresponsible partners.
- The majority of cases of sexually transmitted diseases and HIV/AIDS are the result of destructive sex.
- It is not sanctioned.
- It leads to unwanted pregnancy.
- Pre-marital sex and extra-marital relationships attract calamities that are unforeseeable.
- Real love is replaced by lust of the flesh, which is not strong enough to save a relationship from calamity.
- It damages your soul.

- It is impure.
- It leads to regret.
- It is a perversion of wholesome sex.

> ***An immoral act ends in humiliation; by this act,***
> ***a man is reduced to a crust of bread.***

I have spoken much about immorality and cautioned men against being led into reckless sex by immoral women. In addition, any discussion of destructive sex would not be complete without addressing the issues of incest and sexual assault.

Women and children at risk

Women are often coerced into sexual activities against their wishes. Men are known to make unwanted sexual advances through acts such as misrepresenting their intentions, making crude remarks, pressuring, groping, fondling, and rape. In this way, some men take advantage of their greater physical and social power to exploit women and, even more sadly, children.

Let me state categorically: However a man may choose to justify his actions, any imposed sexual act is a sexual assault, which is forbidden both by the laws of civilized society and by the law of God.

Pressuring a woman by word or action to act contrary to her wishes is wrong. It is a form of cowardice. Rape is an abomination. Incest is an abomination. There are serious consequences to such acts. According to Scripture:

No one is to approach any close relative to have sexual relations. I am the LORD. Do not dishonor your father by having sexual relations with your mother. She is your mother; do not have relations with her. Do not have sexual relations with your father's wife; that would dishonor your father. Do not have sexual relations with your sister, either your father's daughter or your mother's daughter, whether she was born in the same home or elsewhere. Do not have sexual relations with your son's daughter or your daughter's daughter; that would dishonor you. Do not have sexual relations with the daughter of your father's wife, born to your father; she is your sister. Do not have sexual relations with your father's sister; she is your father's close relative. Do not have sexual relations with your mother's sister, because she is your mother's close relative. Do not dishonor your father's brother by approaching his wife to have sexual relations; she is your aunt. Do not have sexual relations with your daughter-in-law. She is your son's wife; do not have relations with her. Do not have sexual relations with your brother's wife; that would dishonor your brother. Do not have sexual relations with both a woman and her daughter. Do not have sexual relations with either her son's daughter or her daughter's daughter; they are her close relatives. That is wickedness. Do not take your wife's sister as a rival wife and have sexual relations with her while your wife is living.[2]

Sexual assault is a perversion and must be abolished. It damages women's sexual life, and many of the victims may forever after find it hard to enjoy a healthy sexual life with their lawful husbands after being assaulted by a relative or a rapist. And frequently, rapists are already HIV-positive.

Let us protect the women in our society by giving no room to sexual assault within the family. We must not allow rapists and child molesters to roam freely on the streets. And women should dress decently to avoid the attraction of a rapist or a lascivious relative or neighbor.

Unfortunately, there are HIV-positive people who intentionally seek to spread the disease, so let us come together to speak out about and stop these atrocious acts. Together we can accomplish this task, because "everything is possible."

Youth at risk: Becoming sexually active to gain approval

Having seen the relationship between sex and HIV, it is really important to emphasize to young people that doing well at school and work should not include sexual immorality. Because schools and

organizations use appraisals to assess scholarly progress and job perfor-
mance and commitment to work, some young people move into sexual
immorality just to get ahead. In the case of young people, ignorance
may be the reason. Here is something for them to consider: *If you
compromise your body for the sake of good grades, you may compromise
your destiny with HIV.* If a grade A+ is the reward for a diligent student
or employee, then grade HIV+ may well be the reward for offering your
body to get ahead. Diligence and God's favor are what it takes to do
well. Your body and soul are at stake, so be careful with anything that
might destroy them. You can win an excellent appraisal without using
your body as an offering.

Social pressure and the need to be accepted can also lead young
people into actions that have unforeseen consequences. In addition to
the danger of getting infected with HIV/AIDS, young people also have
tender hearts that can easily be broken and self-esteem can be damaged.
They often get into situations they are too young to handle, such as
unwanted pregnancies that change their lives forever, no matter how
they decide to handle them.

> **Depending on your actions, you can be appraised
> with a grade A+ or a grade HIV+**

Sexually transmitted diseases (STDs) and HIV/AIDS
What are the sexually transmitted diseases?

They are sexual diseases caused by germs and viruses. They are
contracted mostly through reckless sexual contacts. They are also called
venereal diseases. There are many types of STDs, namely:

- HIV/AIDS
- Candidiasis
- Syphilis
- Gonorrhea

- Pubic lice

- Trichomoniasis

- Genital warts

- Herpes

- Chlamydia

- Chancroids

- Scabies

All the viruses and germs that cause these diseases are found in semen, vaginal fluids, and the blood of an infected person. Some STDs, such as scabies and pubic lice, may be found on the skin or hairs around the genitals. These diseases can only be contracted by having sexual contact with an infected person. Only medical tests or medical examination can indicate that someone is infected with any of these diseases.

STDs can lead to serious health troubles, like itching of the genitals, abdominal pain, and childlessness. To avoid contracting these diseases, we must abstain from sexual immorality. All of these diseases can be cured, except AIDS, which presently has no cure.

Symptoms of STDs

Some common symptoms of sexually transmitted diseases:

- Itching of the genitals

- Pain while urinating

- Abdominal pain

- Genital discharge

- Sore throat

- Skin changes

- Barrenness

- Cancer

- Sores and blisters on the genitals or mouth

It is advisable to seek medical help if you feel uncomfortable or notice an unusual discharge after going to the bathroom.

You can better understand the issue of STDs and HIV/AIDS when you challenge your knowledge of this epidemic by asking yourself questions such as the following. Answer them to your best ability and then read the answers.

How can I tell if I have HIV/AIDS?

The only way to know if you are infected with HIV is to go for a blood test. You cannot rely on symptoms to know whether or not you are infected with HIV. Many people who are infected do not have any symptoms for many years. In addition, the symptoms of AIDS are similar to the symptoms of many other illnesses. If you depend on symptoms, you may wrongly judge your status.

Is there any relationship between HIV and STDs?

More information comes out every day about the link between sexually transmitted diseases (STDs) and HIV. Both HIV and STDs are sexually transmitted through reckless sex: rectal, vaginal, and oral. Consider the following:

- Reckless sex that results in the transmission of an STD also could result in HIV transmission.

- A person with an STD is two to five times more likely to become infected with HIV.

- STDs can cause genital lesions that increase a person's susceptibility to HIV infection.

- A person with both HIV and STD more easily spreads HIV to others.

CHAPTER SIX
ABSTINENCE

Therefore, come out from them and separate yourselves from them, says the Lord. Do not touch their filthy things, and I will welcome you. And I will be your Father and you will be my sons and daughters, says the Lord Almighty. Because we have these promises from the Lord, dear friends, let us cleanse ourselves from everything that can defile our body or spirit. And let us work toward purity because we fear God.[1]

I will start by saying that abstinence is life while pre-marital sex is death.

Abstinence remains the only 100 percent effective means of avoiding HIV/AIDS and other diseases that could be transmitted through sex. Abstaining from sexual relations before marriage and fidelity to your partner in marriage is 100 percent possible.

What is abstinence?

Abstinence means not engaging in sexual activity. When you decide not to engage in sexual activity, it means you are abstaining. In a nutshell, abstinence is running away from sex and all that constitutes sexual behavior.

The majority of young people indulge in sexual activities; only a few abstain. Some avoid intercourse while still engaging in pre-sexual activities, such as kissing, necking, and fondling each other. All these acts are dangerous because they can easily lead to intercourse. Avoid looking at or touching in an unsanctioned way.

Other behavior which most young people today indulge in includes:

- Masturbating
- Watching pornography on the Internet
- Drinking alcohol
- Using drugs of various kinds
- Going out at night unchaperoned or voluntarily being alone with a potential sexual partner or known abuser

All these practices could well destroy your destiny. Do you desire to achieve greatness in life? Do you want to become a doctor, a lawyer, a banker, an economist, an engineer, a pilot, or even the future governor or president? Do you want to be God's ambassador? Then you must run away from every form of unholy behavior that can cut short your desire and cause your soul to perish. Actions such as those I described above easily lead to sexual immorality, which accounts for majority cases of HIV/AIDS, and it is an enemy to your wholesome desires. The only way to achieve what you want in life is to first put your trust in God, run away from all forms of risky behavior, and abstain completely from reckless sex or sex outside of marriage. This is the correct mental disposition of a good citizen and a child of God. You will succeed. Remember, People have chosen this action for centuries, even millennia, so it is possible to adopt this godly lifestyle.

The law of moral excellence

Mary and Joseph before the birth of Christ provide a beautiful model of courtship. Remaining virginal and pure before marriage is a heavenly command. The law of moral excellence requires virtuousness and cleanliness.

Why you should abstain from sexual intercourse outside of a faithful marriage

We have said before that reckless sexual contacts account for the majority of HIV/AIDS cases. If for no other reason, this measure should convince you that it is advisable that sex be restricted to married couples for their enjoyment and for procreation. In other words, men and women must not have sexual relations before marriage and they both must be completely faithful to each other in marriage. Obedience to the law of moral excellence is the best way to protect yourself and your family from HIV/AIDS.

Parents, teach this law to your children. Pass on this message to your families and friends, and you will save many lives.

Young people, you are a source of pride to your parents when you remain pure before marriage. Reckless sex has delivered thousands of lives into the hell of HIV and other STDs and has left millions of people in need of lifesaving treatment. The best ways to avoid being a victim is to abstain from sex before marriage, remain faithful inside of marriage, and avoid sharing objects that can pierce the body. Abstaining from sex before marriage and faithfulness in marriage to your spouse is possible. Everything is possible.

Virginity: a woman's treasure

God honors virginity. To paraphrase from Scripture: Do not despise your youth; conduct yourself in a way that society will respect.[2] If you remain a virgin until you are wed, God will honor and favor you, your parents will respect you, and the wonderful things of life will be compelled towards you. Finally, in marriage, your husband will be extremely favored; as the Scriptures have said, "The man who finds a wife finds a treasure and he receives favor from the Lord."[3] God proclaims a *virtuous woman* an *invaluable treasure* and *a crown to her husband.*[4]

This assertion made me believe that God cherishes virginity and that He expects every virtuous woman to keep her virginity for the appointed time of her favor. That is why the Scripture also says, "There is a time for everything, and a season for every activity under heaven," and "He

[God] has made everything beautiful in its time."[5] This covenant existed before we were born, exists today, and forever remains unbreakable.

Any temptation to lose your virginity before marriage is a temptation to break this covenant, and it may lead you to acquire a killer disease like HIV. Your faithfulness to this covenant has its irrevocable reward. As Scripture tells us, if you diligently obey the voice of the Lord your God and do what is right, He will set you high above all nations of the earth and will bless your bread and water.[6]

A virgin is a precious jewel that cannot be found on the street but must be searched for.

If you remain a virgin, kings will search for you because of your unfathomable values. Be careful with your precious life; your human ability alone cannot win you your highest desire. Only God can put you in the right place at the right time, as was ordained by the Most High long before you became a living creature. Thank God that Mary, the mother of our Lord Jesus, was still a virgin when the time of her favor manifested. If she had not been so, King Emmanuel, the Messiah, would have been born by another virgin. Today, the Lord is saying, "Who is that virgin who will bring my glory to humanity again?" Are you the one?

If your answer is yes, you are blessed among women, and the whole world shall call you blessed. If your answer is no and you are not married, simply ask God to take away the shame of losing your virginity before marriage and forgive you. The Lord will forgive and bless you, as well, but remember that it is always better to be a virgin before marriage. There are numerous blessings in keeping your virginity, because the Lord regards this as obedience, and obedience to the Word of God comes with abundant blessings. As the Scripture says, "If they listen and obey God, then they will be blessed with prosperity throughout their lives. All their years will be pleasant."[7] I have confidence in telling you that a part of what qualifies you as a virtuous woman is your virginity. Keep it, cherish it, and never lose it before marriage. You can get married as a virgin, you can overcome peer pressure, and you can keep your virginity. Every decision can be accomplished because everything is possible.

Some myths about abstinence

Myths are things that many think are true, but which are, in fact, untrue. Do not believe in any of the following myths. They are strategies that friends and others use to corrupt your innocence.

- Abstinence causes pimples.
- Abstinence leads to painful menstruation.
- Abstinence leads to stomach ache due to excess sperm in the male organ.
- Abstinence leads to poor development of the sex organs.
- Abstinence leads to impotence.

Absolutely not! All these myths are lies fabricated to deceive you into indulging in a wrongful act. There are no medical proofs to buttress these assertions. In fact, biological science has taught that:

- Pimples are caused by increased production of oil in the body during puberty and adolescence.
- Development of the sex organs and other physical body characteristics can be traced to one's biological parents.
- Stomachache may be the result of having eaten contaminated food. Visit your doctor.
- Abstinence does not lead to impotence.
- Abstinence is a decent, wholesome, life-saving practice, especially for unmarried people, and it has no negative effects today or tomorrow.

Action formula to help you abstain from sexual intercourse

The best way to abstain from sex is to practice the law of moral excellence. The law of moral excellence requires complete sexual abstinence before marriage and total faithfulness to one's spouse in marriage. This law must become a new chapter of discussion in responsible, Godly families.

- **Dress properly at all times.** Wear clothes that cover your body. Clothes communicate attitude. The way you dress determines how you will be approached.

- **Do not engage in any relationship that demands sexual intimacy as a sign of love.** Your private parts are the pride of your humanity; do not allow anyone to touch them. Do not expose the private parts of your body in public because this might attract a rapist to force you into sex. Most rapists are already HIV/AIDS-positive and are looking for an opportunity to infect other people. Your manner of dressing could attract one today, so dress beautifully and decently.

- **Be decisive.** Your decisions determine your future, which is why you have to be firm in your decisions. No wonder Dr. David Oyedepo* once said that what you have *not* decided cannot be delivered. Examine your mind today to see if you have firmly decided to follow the truth, keep good friends, and abstain from sex. All these decisions have great significance because they constitute the plan of your life. They shape your life, move you towards your dream, and make your destiny a reality. You can achieve only what you have decided to achieve. Every journey in life begins with a decision. It takes courage and decisiveness to abstain from sex outside marriage—no matter the cost, no matter the pressure from your peer group. Your decisions, not the decisions of your friends—will deliver your future. Ignore all bad advice from friends and follow the truth that gives life and saves life. The decision to abstain from sex is one of the most important decisions for your future. Do not just *desire* to abstain from sex, but *decide now* to abstain from sex. Desire alone is not enough.

- **Be disciplined.** For any football team to succeed, every member of the team must be well-trained and disciplined. Self-discipline guarantees success. Discipline is the gateway between goals and accomplishments. All athletes practice strict self-control in order to be winners. You must discipline your body as an athlete does: train it to have the ability to abstain from sex. Only a well-trained and highly disciplined body will be able to abstain from sex. Of course, I realize that "no discipline is enjoyable while it is happening--it is painful. But afterward, there will be a quiet harvest of right living for those who are trained in this way."[8] But remember, self-discipline is not self-punishment. Self-training gives you a better life. The reward of self-discipline is massive divine health and a long, prosperous life.

- **Be determined and focused.** A determined and focused person always secures a place of greatness in life. It takes both determination and focus to completely abstain from sex. Lack of focus is an enemy of destiny. Remain focused, and your destiny will be accomplished.

- **Be a person of integrity.** Integrity safeguards your destiny. Good people are guided by their honesty. Let people know where you stand. For example, Joseph was a man of integrity; he had a blank check to sleep with the wife of his master, but he decided to abstain from sex. Remember, upright citizens bless a city and make it prosper. Say an emphatic *yes* to abstinence, and stand by it no matter how much pressure you are under. In any situation that is contrary to your personal principles and beliefs, always state your position firmly by saying, "No, I can't," or "No, I don't want to."

- **Learn to negotiate.** A negotiation is a discussion that takes place between people of diverse interests in order to arrive at a settlement. It allows people to resolve their conflicts of interest in a mannerly way. Use this ability to negotiate decent and polite relationships that are based totally on mutual respect for everyone involved. Decide what you can and cannot compromise on. Negotiate to abstain from sex if you are in a romantic relationship. The ability to negotiate promotes understanding and protects you from early pregnancy and HIV/AIDS.

- **Learn to communicate skillfully.** Communication is the act of giving, receiving, and understanding messages. It is how you express yourself and your attitude and share information with others. Effective communication will help you talk to people about HIV/AIDS and the reasons for abstaining from sexual activity. Don't be shy. Express your feelings plainly and be an active listener so that you can understand the other person's feelings and respond accurately.

How to say no

You should always refuse any request to do anything you don't want to do by saying no clearly. Make sure your no is a firm no and don't compromise your decision after you have communicated it. Use non-verbal messages like nodding your head or making a gesture to buttress your position. In any circumstance in which you feel you can be exploited or someone wants to take advantage of you, speak out and make your tone of voice strong and audible.

You can say no to requests like the following:

- A request that keeps you from carrying out your daily responsibilities

- A request from anyone—uncle, cousin, friend, sister, brother, acquaintance, and society at large—who is trying to get you to engage in sexual activity, drink alcohol, use drugs, watch sex films, or view pornographic sites on the Internet.

- A request that you should lie in order to party with friends or avoid punishment for something you have done wrong.

- A demand for sex, even if it is just once. A request like this is wrong because even one time puts you in extreme danger of acquiring HIV.

- A request to engage in homosexual activity (male to male sexual relationship). This is unacceptable in the sight of God.

Your body is the temple of God; be careful what you do with it.

- A request to engage in lesbian sexual activity (female to female sexual relationship). This is contrary to the will of God for your life. Live a life and engage in relationships that glorify God.

- In general, any request that seeks to take advantage of you.

Please, always say no to all such requests. They are meant to deceive and distract you from focusing on ABSTINENCE, which is a good way of life.

Follow these steps in refusing a request:

- Simply affirm your position by saying, "No, I cannot do it" or "No, I'm not interested."

- If need be, explain your reasons. For instance, you could say, "It is a sin to engage in sexual intercourse before marriage, and as a child of God, I do not want to commit a sin." Don't feel guilty about your position or standing by your God. It is very simple: just maintain your stand. Godliness exalts a nation, while sin is a disgrace to everyone.[9]

- Always reply immediately to unacceptable requests. Don't say you will think about it or you need some time to reply. It can send a wrong message. It sends a signal that you will change your mind if the person persists. So, it's better to give an instant and firm response.

- Don't ever get into an argument about the issue once you have given your reply. Do not even try to persuade the person to your point of view; just quietly walk away from the scene.

CHAPTER SEVEN
PARENTAL ROLE IN
THE FIGHT AGAINST AIDS

Look, I am going to send you Elijah the prophet before the great and awesome Day of the Lord comes and he will turn the hearts of the fathers to their children and the hearts of children to their fathers. Otherwise I will come and strike the land with a curse.[1]

Parents are faced with one of the most demanding and rewarding tasks in today's civilized world, in which HIV/AIDS is rampant. Successful parenting can only be accomplished through total submission to the will of God and putting your faith on this prophetic promise. We need divine help and divine wisdom, as many forces are battling for the minds and bodies of children as they transition from adolescence to adulthood. It is most essential to rely on God to unite parents and their children in one voice of faith so that the children can obediently embrace the sincere faith of their parents, as was seen in the lineage of Fathers Abraham, Isaac, and Jacob, as well as in the lineage of Lois the grandmother of Timothy, Eunice the mother of Timothy, and Timothy, her son. Lot, the nephew of Father Abraham, and his daughters failed to embrace this sincere faith together, and they equally perished together. This proved to me the Word of God that says, "My people are destroyed for lack of knowledge. Because you have rejected knowledge, I also will reject you from being priest for Me. Because you have forgotten the law of your God, I also will forget your children."[2]

Today, the power of the Holy Spirit is available to unite in holy love the hearts of parents with the hearts of their children. God has placed the responsibility of parenting on the shoulders of the man. Every man or father in a family can be called an Abraham (meaning: 'the father is exalted')[3] by God, and each is to manifest the Abrahamic covenant. "For I have chosen him (Abraham) so that he will command his children and his house after him to keep the way of the LORD by doing what is right and just. This is how the LORD will fulfill to Abraham what He promised him."[4]

God requires that parents not only counsel and advise, but also command that their children and household keep the way of the Lord. God will bestow upon each family and their children who do this the richest manifestation of both spiritual and material blessings. The fulfillment of this promise is not based on the popular song, "Abraham's Blessings Are Mine," but on the capability of Abraham to teach kingdom principles and bring up his children and household in the training and instruction of the Lord. No wonder Pastor E. A. Adeboye said, "The cultivation of basic virtues and proper domestic habits in children is the responsibility of parents." This avowal from this great and exceptional man of God buttresses the assertion that Lot was completely responsible for all the calamities that befell his family.

"For the Lord brought Judah low because of Ahaz king of Israel,
for he had encouraged moral decline in Judah
and had been continually unfaithful to the Lord."[5]

Many parents are dancing to the music of civilization and allowing their children to go astray, dress half naked, dance to corrupt music, and engage in all sorts of compromised behaviors in the name of civilization. Government is not responsible for the moral training of your children; as their parents, you are, and if you fail to domestically infuse core moral values and uprightness into your children, they will conform to what the society can offer them, whether good or bad. Remember, Lot's daughters went against nature, and had unnatural sexual relationships with their father, which was what their society taught them. At times, many parents wonder why their daughters go around half-naked when they themselves do not. But remember the last magazine you took home: no doubt its front page displayed the photo of a half-naked woman. So, young people also read and learn from that. It is high time you put an end to magazines that can lead your daughters astray or teach them things that are contrary to your core values. Your children will reflect the information that is available to them, and they will base their decisions on the knowledge they learn from you or from society.

Parental responsibility

"The rod and rebuke give wisdom,
but a child left to himself brings shame to his mother."[6]

From a Biblical perspective, we can deduce that what children do sometimes might be direct manifestations of what lies in the hearts of their parents or how the parents bring them up. Parents should understand that the family is regarded as the unique department of health, education, and welfare. Children learn more from the example set by their parents than from anything else. Your children might not listen to you all of the time, but they will always copy what you do in their presence. When you are honest, the seed of honesty will germinate and manifest in your children. When you surround them with love, the seed of love will germinate and manifest in them. Children are more likely to remember what they learn by example. What does your child see in you? The answers are best known to you, but please train your children in the ways you know are right. Let them know that choosing the good path is for their utmost benefit. Let us all continually encourage them to fulfill God's plan for their lives. In the words of Scripture, "Teach a child to choose the right path, and when he is older, he will remain upon it."[7]

"The failure of your children points accusing
fingers at your incompetence." — *Pastor E. Adeboye*

The failure of Lot's daughters pointed an accusing finger at Lot, their father. Lot neglected his core responsibility as a father, and his daughters showed their lack of moral values. The fight to defeat HIV/ AIDS must start from our homes; hence, parents must stand up to this responsibility by taking an active role in the education of their children by ensuring that kingdom principles are made active in the family. Monitoring how a child grows up to be a responsible, healthy adult is one of the greatest challenges of parenting, but when parents take an active role, they can meet that challenge by the grace of God. Teens are less likely to have sex at an early age if they are close to parents who clearly communicate strong moral values. The family bond will create an atmosphere of holy love and motivate all family members to discuss tough issues like sex. Children will listen to their parents more than anyone else on these issues. Youth need to be well informed to acquire life skills, such as decision-making, communicating, and negotiating. "And you shall know the truth, and the truth shall make you free."[8] "Sanctify them by Your truth. Your word is truth."[9] The Scripture also tells us, ". . . for You have magnified Your word above all Your name."[10] The Word of God is the principle of God. Sanctify your family today with kingdom principles, and they will reflect the very best and true nature of God.

Your child's health is precious. Do all you can to protect it.

The role of parents in preventing HIV/AIDS

In general, all we have told our children is, "AIDS is real; be careful. AIDS has no cure; be careful." They need to know more. They need to know what AIDS does to the blood and why that is important. They need to understand risky behaviors, such as reckless sex and the use of alcohol and drugs, and the possible consequences of such behaviors. They need to know how to avoid these consequences and where to go for services and help. Every child has a right to the knowledge about how to prevent HIV/AIDS: it could save his or her life.

Building a child's capacity can be gained only in a culture of reading. Brain specialists describe reading as the most valuable tool for brain development. The habit of reading is fast losing ground. Instead, most young people spend their time engaging in unproductive activities, like computer games. The reading habit must be revived and incorporated back into the family norm. Parents must reestablish core moral standards. The Scripture says,

"Train up a child in the way he should go, And when he is old he will not depart from it."[11]

Parents must protect their children; if they do not, who will? We should not allow our children to learn about HIV/AIDS by becoming victims of it. We will be accountable for whatever happens to our children. Give your children the best they deserve. The challenges of the twenty-first century are too enormous to be the sole responsibility of government. Faith-based organizations, corporate organizations, families, individuals, and NGOs must all come together and work together to surmount the many challenges that exist. Together, we can exterminate AIDS. Understanding of AIDS and core moral education will definitely help society to live without AIDS. Everything is possible. Yes, it is possible.

"Indeed, the people are one, and they all have one language, and this is what they begin to do; now nothing that they propose to do will be withheld from them."[12]

Tips for creating a bond within the family

- Set a moral standard on which to build the family's core values. Communicate these values to your children. Write them out and mount them on the wall in their room. This will guide them even while you are not around.

- Ensure that your children are reading literature that will further their education; place such literature where it can easily be seen and read.

- Create a little library or area that encourages young people to study. A little library is better than none at all.

- Parents should be the best examples they can be. Children learn more from them than from anyone else. Charity begins at home. Believe that you are not raising heroes, but are raising sons and daughters, and if you treat them as such, they will turn out to be heroes in your eyes.

- Give your children gifts that are not perishable. Encourage them to always seek more knowledge by reading; remember that readers are leaders.

- Knowledge is the prescription for healing your soul and mind. It will save your life from terrible diseases like HIV/AIDS and give you vibrant hope. Young people should not ignore the vast treasure buried in books.

- Parents should be focused and working on developing strong family ties. Love your spouse, spend excellent time with your family by engaging in recreational activities, and take the family out on holidays if possible. Doing these things will shift your children's minds from immorality and help us all achieve our vision of creating a generation free from HIV/AIDS. Joyful time makes children do well and allows regulation and obedience to seep in.

- A young person regards sex as a leisure activity. Engage your children in more meaningful and acceptable recreational activities that will keep them so busy that they will not have time to discuss or think of sex. Every parent needs to recognize the value of recreation in family life.

- As a matter of urgency, education in morals and in HIV/AIDS should start immediately.

- Teach children to abstain from sex and make sure they practice the law of moral excellence as explained in this book. Correction does much, but encouragement does more. Encourage your child to abstain from sex at all cost.

- When you dream, many wonders can be accomplished. Teach your children to dream big and to aim to achieve the seemingly impossible. They have to have the power and strength from God to achieve whatever they can dream of.

- Your family should pray together regularly. Teach your children how to depend on God and ask Him for all things. Your house should be a mini-church. As it is said, the family that prays together stays together. Teach your children the importance of conducting their lives with diligence.

- Write your children letters or text messages when they are on campus or away at boarding school. Tell them how much you care. Reinforce family values. This practice might seem unworkable, but it works, and it is meaningful if cultivated well.

- Establish core moral standards of sincerity, truth, integrity, honesty, and hard work. These values are the best inheritance you can bestow upon your children; they are better and more valuable than millions of dollars. In fact, they are real income-producing values that will give your family dominion and command.

- By all means, allow your children to have access to youthful liberty, but make sure they do not engage in youthful lusts.

- Read more books on parenting. Remember, your every aim can be accomplished because everything is possible.

The most important things in life are caught and not taught. In other words, children learn more from what they watch you do than from what you teach them. It is essential for parents to fully accept this responsibility, now. As Apostle Paul said to Timothy, "When I call to remembrance the genuine faith that is in you, which dwelt first in your grandmother Lois and your mother Eunice, and I am persuaded is in you also." [13]. Timothy's character was built upon the example first set by his grandmother, Lois, and passed to his biological mother, Eunice. Can this be said about you and your children? We must be their role models. In fact, it is the duty of every parent to emulate Christ. Our children are our best future, our best opportunity, and to us they represent our highest hope, as well. We must not let them down. They are not short-term loans; they are long-term investments. Let's continually encourage them to fulfill God's plan for their lives.

Jesus said, "Let the little children come to me, and do not hinder them, for the kingdom of heaven belongs to such as these."[14] Do not hinder them by your character or your words. Christ greatly delights in doing good for the sake of little children. David, the killer of Goliath, was just a little boy when he became God's choice and was anointed as King. What God saw in David's heart were the core moral values of sincerity, truth, integrity, honesty, and hard work. Apostle Paul saw these same values in young Timothy. Our children can become the best of the best if we give them the best of values. For example, the image a digital camera sees is the image that will print out. Our children will forgive us if we are seen to have tried and failed. But will they forgive us if we fail to try at all?

The image a digital camera sees is the image that will print out.

Abraham trained his children, and he succeeded. Society trained Lot's daughters, and they perished. What kind of father are you? Think about that.

I pray that your sons in their youth will be like well-nurtured plants, and your daughters will be like pillars carved to adorn a palace.

CHAPTER EIGHT
The Role of Youth in Preventing AIDS

"Honor your father and your mother, that your days may be long upon the land which the LORD your God is giving you."[1]

You young people are the future leaders of all nations, and you are also potentially the greatest weapons against HIV/AIDS. You are the joy of your families. God has empowered you with ideas, opinions, and drive to do the right things at the right time. You can build up the capacity to manifest these gifts by honoring God's instructions and learning the right things from role models who guide you correctly. Be the kind of person your parents want you to be. Honor your father and your mother, and your days on earth will be long. Talk to your parents about your beliefs, ideas, opinions, and goals. Let them know what you need from them. Feel free to discuss any issues on which you need more clarification before making significant decisions. Ask your parents questions and talk to them about issues such as HIV/AIDS, relationships, dating, and sexuality. Today's actions will have an impact on your tomorrows.

Tips for kids

Follow with all your heart your family's moral standards and reflect them in your character and decisions.

- Believe that no one is indispensable. Develop your ability to cope with strength and vigor. Engaging in sports, listening to music that will not corrupt your mind, and talking with a helpful, trustworthy adult friend can help you deal with stress.

When you have trusted adults to talk to, you are less likely to use drugs or indulge in unsanctioned sexual activities.

- Be active and eat a healthy diet that regularly includes fruits and vegetables. Participate in enjoyable activities and eat meals with your family as often as possible.

- Be involved in community/faith-based services with your parents. This is a great way to learn responsibility and new skills. It also puts you in touch with other kids who care about people and want to be helpful. Join any volunteer organization in your church or neighborhood that helps people who are living with HIV/AIDS.

- Talk to your parents about your great country. Remember, you are a future leader, and you must let your parents know how you plan to build up the capacity to occupy a leadership position later in life. Learn to understand and respect others. People living with HIV/AIDS are just like everyone else. Like you, they have families and go to school, so show them care and consideration. Playing this important role will showcase your leadership ability.

- Be honest, fair, truthful, and responsible. Be an example that your friends and younger brothers and sisters will follow. Tell the truth and be fair in all your interactions with other kids. If you see that another young person is being treated unfairly, please speak up, and as you do, Almighty God will make you an important person in your generation.

- Maintain an excellent mindset and believe that in the near future, with divine wisdom and understanding, you will solve difficult global problems and, by the power and wisdom of God, provide a cure for HIV/AIDS, which presently is incurable.

- Finally, set yourself apart from destructive influences. Reject all negative influences you know will not provide any value for your life. Such influences may come from your friends or even elderly people. Just avoid being trapped.

You need to remember and believe that you are greatly responsible for what you become in life. God has already given you the power and the grace to subdue obstacles. Building the capacity to attain success in life depends totally on your decision to pursue great things. Your future depends mostly on you. Your capacity, spirituality, and character are the ingredients that will enable you to achieve your God-given victory in life. Never stop reading, never stop dreaming, never stop seeking for righteousness, and never stop seeking information and knowledge, because these things will rouse your inspiration.

Be an active listener. You are born a winner, you are born a leader, you are a born success, and nothing will stop you. The economic situation cannot stop you; the environment cannot stop you. Neither your family background nor your educational background can limit you. Just go a little extra mile in reading, in listening, in seeking righteousness, and in locating information so that your life can become extraordinary.

May you receive God's wisdom and understanding to attain greater height in life. Glory is to God.

New family initiative

The price for a decent society is responsibility. A decent society is possible but the price must be paid by parents who are not just dreaming of a decent society but will take up the responsibility to establish a decent family which can then translated to a decent and better society.

This initiative is an act of imparting your family with generational blessings, and it is also Biblical to sit together as one united family and discuss issues that can prevent family disunity and mishap. The Scripture says, "These words that I am giving you today are to be in your heart. Repeat them to your children. Talk about them when you sit in your house and when you walk along the road, when you lie down and when you get up."[3] Remember Lot didn't follow this Biblical instruction. Lot never used his discretion as a father and his life ended in chaos.

The price for a decent society is responsibility.

"We will not hide these truths from our children but will tell the next generation about the glorious deeds of the LORD. We will tell of his power and the mighty miracles he did. For he issued his decree to Jacob; he gave his law to Israel. He commanded our ancestors to teach them to their children, so the next generation might know them--even the children not yet born. ....[3]. As parents, not hiding these truths from your children is your responsibility

HIV/AIDS discussion within the family

Finally, brethren, whatever things are true, whatever things are noble, whatever things are just, whatever things are pure, whatever things are lovely, whatever things are of good report, if there is any virtue and if there is anything praiseworthy-- meditate on these things.[4]

These are the blessings that God said we should bestow upon our households, but we have neglected religious education for so long that the fearful consequence has been the worldwide outbreak of sexually transmitted diseases, of which some, like HIV, presently have no cure. The statistics of young people between the ages of 15 and 24 who are living with HIV are high, and I do not believe the United Nations or governments alone can turn these statistics around. Parents have an essential obligation to instill the ethics of good conduct in their children. But parents have stopped using their parental authority to restrain their children from bad conduct, and now our streets and cities are filled with professional and corporate prostitutes from reputable homes and schools. Honestly speaking, God is holding parents accountable for this moral decline. Please listen very well: God will judge every home just as He judged Eli's family during Biblical times. Here is what God told Eli: "In that day, I will perform against Eli all that I have spoken concerning his house, from the beginning to the end. For I have told him that I will judge his house forever for the iniquity which he knows, because his sons made themselves vile and HE DID NOT RESTRAIN THEM" (emphasis added).

God is watching over all parents who are not restraining their children from bad conduct and who are hiding the truths from them. He has placed on every parent the responsibility to initiate discussion of core moral values and HIV/AIDS. The more we talk about core moral values and HIV/AIDS, the more we will understand the nature of the disease, and the more lives we will be able to save. It does not matter how much money you have. As a parent, you should have no greater joy than to hear that your children are walking in truth. Create a model to introduce this new initiative in your family today. God is counting on you to use His kingdom principles to enforce the victory at Calvary. In this endeavor, you cannot fail. Sufficiency of power is with you. Every Abraham in every family, everywhere, should step out boldly and start talking about HIV/AIDS and establishing core moral standards of sincerity, truth, integrity, honesty, and hard work. These values are the best inheritance you can give your children. Family values must be built on core moral standards so that we can protect our families, especially our young people, from something that is totally preventable. If you do not protect your families, no one else will. If you think you are not part of the problem, then you cannot be part of the solution. When we own up to our shortcomings, we can find a way to fix them. No matters what happens, a family's moral values become a standard to unite every member of the family.

*The man of the house should take responsibility
for the success and failure of the family.[5] – Ayo Daniels*

Men should not abandon their families because of HIV/AIDS. This would be the most inhumane thing to do. They should avoid pointing an accusing finger at their spouses. It is better to plan the future together, as this increases the hope that can overcome the fear associated with the epidemic. Remember, the future is bright if you take appropriate steps today. You can have a family free from calamity because everything is possible.

CHAPTER NINE
HIV/AIDS, COURTSHIP, AND MARRIAGE

During courtship, practice self-discipline so that HIV does not discipline you. Exert self-control over your body. It may be difficult, but it is not impossible. A courtship that is well-defined and based solely on the eternal principles of God is socially acceptable. Any morally established courtship involves the process by which two believers who intend to become a couple learn more about each other's backgrounds, plan for the future, and sort out their differences. In such a moral relationship, sex is *forbidden*. The forbidden fruit was the means by which sin entered into human nature, and today, sex during courtship is the major gateway through which HIV/AIDS enters human blood. Partaking of any forbidden fruit has severe consequences and must always be avoided.

It is a fallacy to believe that sex before marriage is a proof of potency. Everyone born of God has the replenishing and fruitful nature of God; everyone is naturally endowed with the supernatural strength and capacity to multiply. Potency is not based on your physical ability to have sex; it is a gift from the Omnipotent God. In fact, only God, who owns creative power, has the gift of potency. Only God, who has sufficiency of power, can make everything possible.

"None of your men or women will be childless[1] . . .
The smallest family will multiply into a large clan.
The tiniest group will become a mighty nation. I, the LORD,
will bring it all to pass at the right time."[2]

This is the unchangeable eternal truth that confirms the gift of potency from God. Sex has its proper time for the fulfillment of God's purpose for marriage. Intending couples must bide their time and not engage in sex until marriage, because every shortcut in life can cut down your life. Every instance of sex before marriage is a shortcut; it may lead to HIV, and HIV cuts down people's lives.

It is a mere speculation that makes people believe that sex before marriage is the cure for barrenness. This is just human perception. It is in God's nature to make our families as plentiful as the grains of sand on a beach. This truth is unchangeable, everlasting, and settles the fact that none among us shall be barren because *"The Strength of Israel will not lie"*

> *"So put to death the sinful, earthly things lurking within you.*
> *Have nothing to do with sexual sin, impurity, lust,*
> *and shameful desires. Do not be greedy for the good things*
> *of this life, for that is idolatry. God's terrible anger will come*
> *upon those who do such things."*[3]

Do not be deceived; there is no moral justification for sex before marriage. Sex before marriage is the fastest means of acquiring HIV/ AIDS. This is an opportunity for you to stay clean and live right. Start living correctly now; don't wait until tomorrow. If you think you can indulge one more time before you stop, you might not survive the next act. You can stop now by living right and disciplining yourself.

Again, it is important to know that courtship should be established only between two believers, because God has instructed us never to team up with those who are unbelievers. How can piety be a partner with impiety? How can light live with darkness? What harmony can there be between Christ and the devil? How can a believer be a partner with an unbeliever? The Scripture says "Do not be unequally yoked together with unbelievers. For what fellowship has righteousness with lawlessness?" And what communion has light with darkness (See 2 Corinthians 6:14.) Do not ever think you can change unbelievers by entering into a relationship with them. Allow God to change them before you ever think of establishing any permanent relationship with them. They might corrupt your faith or lead you into the trap of sexual immorality. Many believers have been led into wrongdoing based on this assumption, and today many more are still under the influence of the devil; thank God, your story is different, because He that lives in you is greater than Satan and his foolish devices.

Scripture tells us that Satan is a condemned being. "A good man obtains favor from the Lord, but a man of wicked intentions He will condemn."[4] Any time Satan puts a wrong idea into your mind, just tell him, "Old boy, you are a condemned man, and I am not your candidate, so just maintain a distance." As you declare this, Satan has no other option but to run away from you, because he does not want to hear the truth. Only the truth can make Satan flee back to his constituency of darkness, because the truth is too acidic for him to bear.

> *Sexual immorality is like a pothole on the road*
> *that leads to marital destruction.*

We are all familiar with the potholes on our paths. They have cut short many journeys, just as sexual immorality can cut short destiny. You must be faithful to God and to yourself to achieve your rightful destiny. When a car repeatedly drives over potholes, gradually the shock absorbers, the tires, the wheel rims, and other vital parts of the car are worn down. If we fall into sexual immorality, we are gradually destroying our precious destiny. Remember, there is no condom that protects the soul and your rightful destiny.

HIV/AIDS and marriage

Just before you say, "I do," take an HIV test so that both of you will know your HIV status, and ever after remain faithful to your partner.

> *Let your "Yes, I do" be only to your spouse.*

I can do all things through Christ who strengthens.[5] "Yes, I do" means that with the strength of Christ, you will remain faithful. The moment you do otherwise, you are inviting family misfortune. Therefore, just remain faithful to your God-given partner. Every unfaithful union or extramarital relationship invites incurable diseases like HIV/AIDS and other sexually transmitted diseases. You must be unerringly faithful, honest, and sexually responsible at home. These three ingredients are the prerequisites to a successful marriage and a family free from the scourge of HIV/AIDS and other STDs. Be careful with your life; the costs of infidelity are greater than the benefits, and only a foolish person would follow this pathway.

You wives must submit to your husbands, as is fitting for those who belong to the Lord. And you husbands must love your wives and never treat them harshly.[6]

You husbands must give honor to your wives.
Treat her with understanding as you live together.
She may be weaker than you are.[7]

Let the Holy Spirit control your lives and guide you into all truth so that He can produce the fruit of love, peace, patience, kindness, goodness, faithfulness, gentleness, and self-control.[8] With these, you will experience heavenly blessings, a healthy relationship, and one united family without the fear of acquiring HIV/AIDS. Dwelling together in unity is a heavenly command: do not depart from it.

Looking for assistance or support in the wrong places

Looking for support in the wrong places has led many to seek out different sexual partners. This is a common practice in our places of work and on our campuses. Ladies depend on their male counterparts for material gain, promotion, and financial rewards. As a result, they may enter into sexual relationships with men who can benefit them materially. Such men, too, take pride in being involved with several women. It is not an achievement when you have several sexual partners; rather, it is a symptom of coarseness, waywardness, or lust. Such irresponsible attitudes can gradually destroy your future. In fact, looking for help where it cannot be found is labor lost.

"Therefore let no one boast in men. For all things are yours."⁹

Only God can help. All things you need to fulfill your rightful destiny are yours and have been given to you. The talent, the wisdom, the boldness, the creativity, the courage, the determination, and the capacity—all are wrapped up in your inner pocket. Look up to God for the manifestation of your gift, not to a person. Let no man glory in others, for all things are yours in Christ. Know that your sufficiency is from God. That is why you will excel in every good work you do, because "everything is possible."

What you do today can save your future tomorrow. Remain faithful to your partner if you are already married and abstain from sex if you are still single. Look to God for help, promotion, provision, and security, because He is the only one who can supply all your needs.

CHAPTER TEN
The Cure for Hopelessness

This is a call to choose hope over fear. HIV is no longer a death sentence. There are treatments and antiretroviral medications that can suppress the virus and prevent or decrease your symptoms. Living with HIV/AIDS does not mean that you must stop dreaming or allow depression to overcome you. HIV/AIDS should be viewed like any other disease; it does not have the power to stop your dreams and visions. Direct every vision to adding value to others. Do this so that your vision is not about yourself alone, but also a mission to help your generation.

Every situation can be a turnaround, a new beginning, and a sign of unending passion for your vision.

Being HIV/AIDS-positive does not make you medically unfit to achieve your vision; you still can live positively and fulfill your vision to become your best. HIV/AIDS-positive people can and do create wealth, have jobs and careers, win national appointments, and become the leaders of tomorrow. Your rights are equal to those of every other person in the world. Work diligently at your dream, and you can be certain of great and mighty success.

HIV does not kill your vision, but lack of knowledge can send you into captivity. Your limitations and achievement today are a direct function and clear reflection of your knowledge or lack of it. With the right kind of knowledge, you can always be greater and better than you are presently. Always seek for knowledge, because knowledge brings awareness. Knowledge fights the ignorance in you and makes you aware of every opportunity that arises. It awakens you by turning on your inner light. Knowledge brings you full understanding.

Hopelessness can strike anyone, whether he or she is HIV/AIDS-positive or -negative, and hopelessness can kill you faster. Even so, people living with HIV may be at greater risk for depression, which can make you weak in both body and mind. Depression affects how you relate to the people around you, and if left untreated, can cause a relationship to deteriorate. Some people respond to depression by becoming angry with or abusive to people who care about them or children who depend on them. Others react by taking alcohol or hard drugs in an attempt to suppress depression, but this will only quicken HIV's progression to AIDS. Cultivating maximum hope can help to overcome depression and fight against HIV/AIDS, and this will enable you to live longer.

Winning in life is not just sitting down and figuring out the equations; rather, it requires diligently working toward your vision with a positive attitude. Vision gives you hope; it is the cloth that every destiny is made of; vision is the art of making what appears to be impossible, possible. Be proud and be responsible. Change your mindset and live positively to achieve your dreams in life.

My candid advice to all young people is that you should never gamble with your future. Total abstinence remains the surest means to protect yourself from HIV/AIDS. Remember, abstinence includes refusing to look at anything that is forbidden. Do not set before your eyes anything that is worthless and that can destroy you. Abstinence is the only real preventive medicine for HIV/AIDS. You will succeed.

Having HIV is not the end of your dreams or the end of your journey; it is just an opportunity to look at life from another perspective. Just like Solomon, having thought about life from a deep place, said, "Vanity of vanities; all is vanity."[1] If you are conscious of the power inside, you can fulfill your future. Then the issues of living with HIV will become part of you and you can realize that a miracle from God can remove it at any time. In the kingdom of God, there is no such thing as speculation--God is God, He does not change and all things are possible with Him.

No matter what situation you are confronted with, you can overcome hopelessness, because you are born of God, and anyone who is born of God is an overcomer. *Put your trust in God* by meditating on "whatever things are true, whatever things are noble, whatever things are just, whatever things are pure, [and] whatever things are lovely."[2] Talk about things that are excellent and worthy of praise. This will give you a positive mind-set which provides the energy for a successful life. If you are already a victim of HIV, CONTINUE with your treatment, visit your medical professional in a timely manner, and above all, do not stop praying to God.

Prayer can change anything.

I am sure the yoke of HIV shall be destroyed because of the anointing of Christ in your life. Now I am encouraging you to choose hope over fear and get pregnant with the Word of God, and your healing will manifest.

A positive mindset provides the energy for a successful life.

Hopelessness gives you a negative mindset and causes you to give up. Although having HIV or wasting disease may be a bitter pill to swallow, much good is in you, and I am confident that with God all things are possible. So, right now, start living with the consciousness that "everything is possible." For instance, the best wisdom of science has only been able to construct bridges over the sea, but God alone has parted the sea. Jesus is that bridge. I am confident that this same God who has been, is, and will be the same yesterday, today, and forever, will work through your situation right now and wipe out the handwriting of ordinances against you, in the name of Jesus. There is a compelling force in the name of Jesus that subdues every other name. Beginning right now, stop calling this disease HIV/AIDS; that is the language of the world; instead, call it *wasting disease*, as it is written in the Bible. The source of your life depends only upon the victory of Christ. There is undeniable victory in the name of Jesus; there is unquestionable victory in the name of Jesus; there is incontestable victory in the name of Jesus. In the mighty name of Jesus, I decree that every depression and wasting disease is over.

The value of hope

Cultivating hopefulness may improve your way of thinking and give you the spiritual strength to face your entire situation as it comes.

Hope can help you fight against HIV/AIDS, and this will enable you to hold the positive beliefs.

- You may live for many years.
- A cure may be found very soon.
- God will cure you if you pray and cultivate holiness.
- "Everything is possible."

CHAPTER ELEVEN
LASTING GLOBAL SOLUTION
TO DEFEAT AIDS

If you think morality is a luxury business can't afford,
try living in a world without it
—*Anita Roddick, Founder and Co-Chair, The Body Shop[1]*

As an economist, I love to analyze a problem so that I can apply a well-detailed solution. In my private research and analysis on this global epidemic, I discovered that HIV/AIDS is *not* a contagious disease and that the major cause of HIV/AIDS in the world today is *immorality*. A world without morality is full of shame and the reproaches of HIV/AIDS. A family or life without morality is full of discomfort and dishonor. HIV/AIDS is a moral issue, and it needs a moral solution. Immorality paves the way for HIV/AIDS, a life-destroying infection. AIDS is one of the by-products of immorality. AIDS presently has no cure, but immorality can be cured, defeated, or corrected. Immorality can be turned into morality. Do not wait until immorality takes over the whole world. At home and at school, we can no longer fold our arms and allow it to destroy the lives of our youth.

The global solution to defeat AIDS begins with you; don't refer your responsibility to government or the United Nations. It is up to you and me to lay a moral foundation for our youth and the next generation. We cannot afford to wait until HIV/AIDS destroys the lives of young people; let us start the fight now. A world full of morality can exterminate AIDS; morality can stamp out AIDS; let's spread kingdom principles to others around us. Together, we can win the fight against AIDS. Remember, everything is possible. Yes, it is.

Immorality begets AIDS.

Biblical history gives us the knowledge that the ancient people acquired a wasting (killer) disease through acts of sexual immorality and that twenty-four thousand people died as a result of the epidemic; today, thousands are dying daily as a result of HIV/AIDS. It would be advisable for us all to learn from Biblical history, because the vast majority of cases of HIV/AIDS are acquired through sexual immorality. These two assertions clearly establish the reality that immorality begets HIV/AIDS (killer diseases). Our major assignment is to defeat HIV/AIDS in our communities, our society, and the world by fighting ignorance and immorality, which are the genesis of HIV. If we do not do this, fighting HIV/AIDS is just a mirage. People indulge in immorality because they are ignorant of its consequences and they lack moral values.

Thinking that we can defeat HIV/AIDS on the street is a misconception. This can never be achieved until we collectively, as families, communicate strong values to children and thereby uproot the ignorance and immorality which beget HIV/AIDS. God has instructed us to commit ourselves wholeheartedly to His commands and to repeat them again and again to our children, both at home and in school. Today, immorality is everywhere just because both parents and teachers have failed to do this. Parents have neglected this responsibility and it has been said that *the price for a decent society is responsibility*. If we are to drive out immorality and create a generation free from HIV/AIDS, the gears of our vehicles must always be on morality, which can then translate into successful achievement of the objectives contained in the United Nations Millennium Goals. When we uproot our society's immorality, then to a great extent we will have uprooted HIV/AIDS out of that same society. AIDS presently has no cure, but immorality does. When youth are conscious of moral values, they will find it shameful to enter into immoral activities.

What our children need most are not thousands of shares in stock but guided moral fiber.

To fight immorality, we must fight in its totality whatever draws the eyes of the young people into immorality, which includes not only pornography but also poverty mentality. Scripture tells us, "The lamp of the body is the eye. If therefore your eye is good, your whole body will be full of light. But if your eye is bad, your body will be full of darkness . . ."[2] Apart from giving us the ability to see, the eye conveys expression and reveals our inner disposition. What you set your eyes upon goes into your mind and will control your body. That is why Scripture tells us not to look at anything that is vile and vulgar. Pornographic websites and magazines are vulgar and corrupting and should be restricted.

Our manner of dress matters. Clothes may look beautiful, but not be decent. Beautiful clothes that look sloppy and provocative are not decent. Some brag that a provocative outfit was half-price, but if truth be told, half of it is also missing. Teach your young people to always dress in decent clothes that are both beautiful and presentable. We must also tell young people that lack of material wealth does not translate into being poor. We must change this mentality. Our youth need a new mindset, and they must also be taught to be creative and productive by using their inner strengths to create genuine wealth. God has given each and every one of us the power to become rich and live like champions. As a popular saying goes, "Everyone may have been born naked on the outside but no one is born empty on the inside." Everyone is born with a unique gift to take him or her to the mountaintop. You are meant to make an impact on the world with your gift. God did not put your success in the hands of anyone else. What will take you to the zenith of life is hidden inside you, and no one can lay claim to it except *you*. You are exceptionally important to this world; no other person can be you or occupy your place. Discovering your gift is what will set you on the road to *greatness*.

This is the new mindset you must have. This new mindset will set you apart for greatness, which is your *birthright*. This new mindset will create in you the joy of living a moral life, and a moral life circumvents AIDS.

The salt in you is your gift.

In my opinion, our world needs a revival of *genuine moral uprightness*. Just as much as the military is concerned about developing guided missiles to prevent the deaths of innocent people during a conflict, parents and the world should be even more concerned about guided moral character to avoid and defeat this deadly disease known as HIV/AIDS. Parents should not just pray alone, they should start acting now and getting involved in shaping the world into a new configuration that is totally free from HIV/AIDS.

At this defining moment in history, our individual actions are what count towards defeating the world's most dreadful disease. Let us send a powerful message that the world was created by God and belongs to God, and God alone is the Father of morality and possibility. I have decided to give my best to beautify the world in my own capacity through Christ. If this is the mental disposition of everyone in the world, we will make the world more habitable for the next generation. Do your part today to save our world. Immorality cannot defile the armies of God.

The forty-third president of United States, George W. Bush, once asked the Congress in 2003 to commit $15 billion dollars to turn the tide against AIDS in the most afflicted nations of Africa and the Caribbean. More nations keep donating to fight this epidemic yet it is on the increase. With this, I believe that these efforts will give us a positive result if they are complimented by a high standard of moral living in the family, because a *moral life circumvents AIDS*.

Believe that *a moral life circumvents AIDS,* and remember that you are the solution. Do not go back to bed and sleep when you need to proffer a solution to the world's problems. You can have whatever you desire; no dream is too big to be accomplished. If you believe you can, you will. *Everything is possible.*

CHAPTER TWELVE
LIVING A LIFE OF MORAL EXCELLENCE FREE OF AIDS

A life of moral excellence without HIV/AIDS is possible.
"Everything is possible."

HIV/AIDS, in most cases, is a product of lack of discipline, lack of self-control, and immorality. A life of moral excellence is a product of your faith, which is why the Scripture tells us, "A life of moral excellence leads to knowing God better. Knowing God leads to self-control. Self-control leads to patient endurance, and patient endurance leads to godliness. Godliness leads to love for other Christians, and finally you will grow to have genuine love for everyone."[1] The more you grow and work in these ways, the more your life will become creative and practical through your knowledge of our Lord Jesus Christ. A creative and practical life is a life of distinction and focus; only a life that is focused on moral excellence is guaranteed to be free of AIDS. A life of moral excellence is a life dedicated to God, and whatever you dedicate to God will manifest the glory of God.

If your mental disposition as a child of God is to live a life of moral excellence, then you are born to excel and win. A winner is someone who fulfils his or her life purpose. You must have a creative mind to succeed in this present world.

There are immoral, worldly ways in which we can reap quick financial benefits, but such financial benefits have resulted in calamity upon calamity. Unfortunately, our minds have been programmed since we were born to think in terms of scarcity. We grew up in the midst of an economic theory rooted in the perception that resources are scarce or inadequate, and fighting for scarce resources has led many into committing immoral acts. Now, many people take abnormal steps to acquire these perceived limited resources at the expense of their fellow citizens.

Now, we need to reprogram the mind with what the Creator of the universe said, ". . . if you consent and obey, you will eat the best from the land."[2] How? By being diligent and cultivating a new mindset, you will be able to create something exceptional out of the scarcity of the earth that no economic theory would be able to explain. For instance, no economic theory in the world can explain how our Lord Jesus, by looking up to heaven, fed a multitude with just five loaves of bread and two fish. It was a manifestation of the inexplicable grace of God, which long before our birth made it possible for all creatures to manifest with both signs and wonders.

You are just a mortal body, but God breathed on you, and this breath is the *breath of life*; this breath quickens your mortal body and sets every part into motion. This breath inspires the creative ability in you to come forth. This is why the Scripture tells us that you are an exceptional being who is "fearfully and wonderfully made."[3] You cannot fail because you are *God-master builder*. There is something in you that will change the face of your world. The Superlative Intelligence made you the salt of the world and you must add value and preserve this world. *Mother Teresa* is an example of those who added value to humanity. I have never heard how much money she left in her bank account, but I have heard how many lives she affected. She made history because of her contribution to her generation. You can reshape what she did in another form. This is why the Scriptures say that the world is waiting for your manifestation. She was a winner and an accomplisher because, even today, the world still reveres her good works. You can equally be a winner and an accomplisher by simply focusing on what you can contribute to society rather than on what you can get. Your contribution to society is what determines your accomplishment.

Your contribution determines your achievement.

Winners are committed thinkers! Thinking brings understanding, and a man of understanding will be outstanding. The ability to think is your access to living an outstanding life. What you have not thought about cannot be delivered to you. Thinking is the most productive and least energetic activity I have ever known. Engaging your mind in productive thinking does not require any extra energy other than the ability to remain tranquil. The ability to think gives you the capacity to see things that do not exist as if they do. Thinking is the ability that allows you to imagine how to do things in better ways. In fact, you are a product of your thinking. Thinking is the ability to change scarcity into abundance. *If you can imagine the unimaginable, you can do the undoable. Everything is possible.*

Your mind is a satellite that can comprehend great things before they physically happen.

There is a connection between your mind, your brain, and your success. Success begins from your mind. Thinking and meditation take place in your mind. A peaceful mind generates a powerful mental attitude. Success is the ability to think and to imagine possibilities even for what on the surface appears unworkable; you need to speak of what is possible as if it were already accomplished. It would be correct to say that divine success is a result of positive thinking and positive action. Remember, good thinking produces a good product. *If you can think it, you can create it.* Success is discernible in prayer, but it is attainable through action

Thinking repositions your mind to conceive creative ideas.

Therefore, to achieve divine success, you must combine your thoughts and your actions. Thought provides a mental picture of your desire, and you receive your desire through action. The mental disposition of a child of God is what it takes to live a life of moral excellence without AIDS.

The Almighty's formula for success

As discussed in the previous chapter, many people look in the wrong direction for help, and this has resulted in HIV/AIDS. Looking up to God has its own price tags and rewards, as well. The Scripture gives us the Almighty's formula for success:

> *Ask, and it will be given to you;*
> *Seek, and you will find;*
> *Knock, and it will be opened to you.*[4]

The price tags are *Ask, Seek,* and *Knock,* while the rewards are *you will be given, you will find,* and *it will be opened to you.* The price tags are the actions you personally take to look up to God for help, and the rewards come from God's unchangeable covenant that He is ready to fulfill. Scripture says, "Those who look up to him [God] for help will be radiant with joy; no shadow of shame will darken their faces."[5] If you stay outside of God's commands or allow yourself to be derailed from them, you will miss your way; but if you remain in God, you can do everything. According to Scripture, "Even more blessed are all who hear the word of God and put it into practice."[6]

How you can put the Almighty's formula into practice and be more blessed

- Ask

How do you ask from God? Scripture tells us, "Call to Me, and I will answer you, and show you great and mighty things, which you do not know."[7] This does mean you should complain. Put a smile on your face. Isaiah 12:3 says you shall, with joy, draw water from the wells of salvation. Speak in understanding and in tongues, and at the end of the call, tell God you love Him. He will respond, "But I first loved you." The Scripture says, "We love Him because He first loved us."[8] As you remain joyful in prayer, the light of God will come upon you like a revelation. According to the words of Scripture, ". . . all these blessings shall come upon you and overtake you."[9] A revelation is an eye-opener to God's secret plan for you.

- **Seek**

The second line says, "Seek and you will find." It means that you need to sit down and ponder the revelation God has given you. Search your inner mind; meditate over that revelation. Look around you and relate this revelation to something practical, like your gift. Paint a clear and definite mental picture of what you want or what the revelation tells you. Form a mental picture of the possibilities in this revelation. Think big about the revelation. Discover your potential as you meditate on it. Feel worthwhile about yourself. See the possibilities in it.

Whatever enters your mind and occupies your thoughts has the capacity to deliver to you your destiny. Do not entertain any negativity. Holding this great mental picture in your mind, begin to direct your attention towards what you desire. Retain this clear mental picture, just as a pilot holds the mental picture of the airport at which he intends to land.

> *What you can defeat in your mind has no power*
> *to oppress you in the physical.*

You must see that the manifestation of that mental picture is possible before you can deliver it. Cultivate a peaceful mind. A peaceful mind generates unimaginable power for overcoming obstacles. What you can defeat in your mind has no power to oppress you in the physical. You can alter your life by altering your thought processes. Quietude is the appointed time during which great things and great opportunities are returned to you as newer and bigger opportunities. Expect the best in every situation. As you begin to think in this manner, you are building up your faith, and remember, *it will be unto you according to your faith; if your faith can see everything, you can have everything.*

• **Knock**

The third line of this Scripture says, "Knock and it will be opened to you." Before we go further, let us ask ourselves this question: When, as a visitor, you arrive at the door, what do you do? Do you just stand there, or do you knock to signify your arrival? If you just stand there without doing anything, no one will know you are there. When you knock, someone is likely to respond. Your action provokes a response. Science has indicated that action and reaction are equal and opposite. To get a reaction, you have to act, in our example, the action is to raise your hand and knock. Knocking at the door causes it to be opened unto you. The great and effective doors of God do not open until you take action. Remember, success is discernible in prayer but attainable by action.

Knocking at God's door means taking practical steps to act on God's Word. The answer will bring abundance. Like a tree planted along the riverbank, you will bear fruit in each season, without ceasing. Your leaves will never wither, and in everything you do, you will prosper.[10] So don't just stand there, looking and hoping that things will take their proper shapes without putting forth any effort. Put your faith to work; act on His revelation.

How many of us are just standing here and looking at God's revelation without taking any steps to actualize it? Action taken with faith is what separates a winner from a loser. A winner will always act on God's Word, while a loser takes no action. The Bible says,

"Do you see a man skilled in his work? He will stand in the presence of kings."[11] Embrace the concept of hard work.

How many of us are not acting on the potential God deposited in us? Our potential is God's endowment within us to ensure that we have divine success in life. John C. Maxwell said, "One of the greatest days of your life will be the day when you discover your potential."[12] God knew you before you were born; at birth, He deposited something of great value in you that the whole world cannot ignore. Meditate on God's Word day and night. Abide by all that has been revealed to you. A winner is full of God's wisdom, because wisdom is what compels you to act on the Word of God. Abiding by this third line, *knocking*, is what establishes your faith and belief in God. Dear brothers and sisters, what is the use of having faith if you do not prove it by your action? Faith without action is useless.[13] No matter how big your dream and how vivid your mental picture, no matter how good and realistic it seems, it will remain only a dream unless you take the necessary action to actualize it—today.

Success is discernible in prayer but attainable by action.

Subject the revelation God has given you into intensive thinking. Understanding will come of it, and then victory will be certain. *When you think enough, you will succeed more than enough.* Stop speculating; divine success in life does not come by speculating but from God's revelation. Rick Warren said, "Revelation beats speculation any day."[14] As an economist, I know the power of speculation in the money market, especially when you have accurate data to work with. However, there is a limit to the success that speculation can produce, because of the variability and inconsistency of data. Speculation can produce failure as well as success.

God's revelation is eternal truth. It is consistent, it is unchangeable, it is predictable, it is constant, and it is current. It is an unbreakable covenant that can only produce divine success and never produces failure. The product of God's revelation is divine success; it is knowable, and it is everlasting in nature. Good thinking combined with right action equals divine favor, and favor is what takes you to the right place at the right time. On the other hand, bad thinking with right action equals earthly success, and we know that earthly success has no lasting value. God's royal decrees cannot be changed.

When you think enough, you will succeed more than enough.

The Scripture says, "As he [a man] thinks in his heart, so is he."[15]

If a man thinks in his mind that everything is possible, so it is. That is why the Scripture says we should fix our thoughts on what is true, honorable, and right; think about things that are pure, lovely, and admirable; and think about things that are excellent and worthy of praise.[16]

By thought, you can cause the riches in the heart of a lion to come forth, but the lion will not just vomit them up. You have to take the uncompromising step of killing the lion. In other words, your thoughts must connect to personal action. Set your heart on the eternal truth. Negative thought never produces success. Negative thought is the enemy's strategy to steal the word of God from your heart and make you think God has forgotten you. God cares about you more than you know. For instance, the former generation of people ate manna from God for forty years, but His covenant with us as a later generation is everlasting manna, and our new manna as believers under this new covenant is the grace of God, which is infinite.

Those who receive the abundant grace of God shall reign in life.

The grace of God is the only thing that will set you apart in your endeavors. All obstacles to your destiny are overwhelmed by the grace of God. His grace is abundantly available to you. You cannot do anything to merit it; God gives it to you irrespective of your age, gender, and location so that you may have divine victory.

- We understand that God's Word teaches us that grace is free and undeserved. To show the effectiveness of God's grace in your life, embark on your big dream, and make sure this dream is directed at adding value to people's lives; ensure that this dream is more than your ability. Then you will see God at work on your behalf.

- God's grace as the divine manna from heaven should make you start taking gradual steps towards realizing your dream. The bigger your dream, the bigger the grace of God you attract. *Like attracts like and deep calleth unto deep*

As the Scripture clearly says, "By strength shall no man prevail [succeed, triumph, overcome, and reign]."[17] What it means is that human strength will fail us. We all need to depend on the grace of God as the banner of strength and the power to attain the best of our dreams.

Change your mental habits, focus on God's Word, and expect the best: expect great things; expect divine success and long life. What you expect is what you get. "And we know that all things work together for good to those who love God, to those who are the called according to His purpose."[18]

You have been made a king, and the Word of God says, "The king's command is backed by great power. No one can resist or question it."[19] When you decree a thing in the name of Jesus, so shall it be, because those who receive abundance of grace shall reign in life. Do not just sit down. Stand up, take action, enjoy God's grace, and start reigning like a king. Your thought is the genesis of magnification; what will take you to the highest level in life is your thinking pattern, and whatever you can defeat in your mind has no power to oppress you in the physical.

Doing something about God's word

God's revelation is like an international treaty in which every country that is a party to the treaty must play her role to make sure it works by abiding by the terms of the treaty. When God gives out a revelation, it is always between God and you. He has His unbreakable covenant to keep, and we have our responsibilities to play as well. God is committed to His covenant. For the integrity of His holy name, we will enjoy His covenant of giving us divine success. When God gives you a seed, He expects you to plant it. The Bible says, *"The hand of a diligent man will rule."*[20] Embrace the concept of hard work. It pays and its rewards are excellent.

When God gives you a revelation or a vision, He expects you to meditate on it and to diligently act according to all that you have seen. This will assure you divine success. Diligence attracts divine grace, and the key to success is the grace of God. Pursue it, and you will succeed in life, in the name of Jesus. Amen.

Divine purpose

Greatness is God's divine purpose for your life.

This statement is talking about you; even as an embryo in your mother's womb, you were already a finished vision. God created you for greatness. God had His divine purpose, and He created you to fulfill that purpose. Greatness is the divine purpose of God for your life. You are born to accomplish something specific that the whole world cannot disregard, something that can make you unforgettable, something that only you can deliver. The answer to the world problem is in your spirit. This generation and the next are counting on you. Success is in your spirit; you are programmed to succeed. There is more to your life than your physical appearance or your present status. Therefore, "Whatever your hand finds to do, do it with all your might."[21] Success beyond measure awaits you as you take bold action toward the attainment of your dream. Remember, everything is possible.

You cannot achieve greatness unless you discover its access route.

There is a road that leads to achieving the divine purpose of God for your life. The divine purpose of Jesus Christ is to lay and establish the foundation for the expansion of God's kingdom. That is why we refer to Christ as the greatest. He went to the cross and was sent back to be our helper (as the Holy Ghost), to help us build on the foundation

He laid in expanding God's kingdom. That means we can only achieve greatness by focusing on the expansion of God's kingdom which is the access route to greatness.

What vehicle can we drive on the divine road?

Now that we know the road to unfolding God's divine purpose, earthly vehicles cannot move on it, because they cannot produce the friction needed to make them road-compliant. If you try to use earthly vehicles to travel the divine road, you will struggle and never succeed. It is a road created by God, and only vehicles created by God can generate the required friction to travel without breakdowns, pothole damage, and other malfunctions. Even without fuel, God's vehicle will move on this road. Without headlights, it will move on this road, because the driver of this vehicle is the Light of the world. Without gear, this vehicle will move on this road. Just a contact with the driver will jump-start all the divine requirements to get the vehicle moving. God's vehicle is invisible, yet it is better than the most sophisticated earthly vehicle. When you discover and develop it, it will take you to the top faster, because its speedometer is divine and unbreakable.

How do you discover and develop this vehicle?

"Upon this rock I will build my church,
and all the power of hell will not conquer it."[22]

What is the rock spoken of in the above Biblical quote? *Self-discovery.* Self-discovery is the starting point for all great achievers in the kingdom of the Most High God. It means knowing who you are through God's revelation and what you were born to fulfill. The best way to discover yourself is to dedicate your time to studying, meditating, and praying on the Word of God, which is like a mighty hammer that smashes a rock to pieces. Only the Word of God can reveal to you who you are and what you were born to fulfill. The Word of God will make you to discover what is within you, what God has placed in your inner pocket.

If you look within yourself, you will find a treasure. The gift deposited in you will unlock all doors to your greatness in life. Developing your gift makes possible you doing great things. A man's gift will bring him before important people.

For instance, in the entertainment industry, comedians used to be nobody, but today the creative minds of these people are paying off heavily. They crack jokes and they get paid fairly well. Just by working on their minds and developing their potential to turn real-life situations into humor, they have become known for this gift and the world celebrates them. No wonder Dr. Myles Munroe said, "Whenever you exercise your gift . . . the world will not only make room for you, but it will also pay you for it."[23] It is time for you to start using your inner strength to compel the attention of the universe towards your life. Do not just sit there. Be diligent. Take up your gift, and it will make a way for you. It will turn you into an overnight star. "Everything is possible."

Only a divine vehicle can work on a divine road to reach a divine destination. Your divine destination is greatness; greatness is God's divine purpose for your life, and God's divine purpose is the expansion of His kingdom on earth. It is our responsibility to use our divine vehicle.

Only the Greatest Teacher can show you the way to your greatness.

The day you accept Christ into your life, a certificate of greatness is placed in your hands, and your responsibility is to manifest what is written on the certificate. That is why the Scripture states, "The earnest expectation of the creation eagerly waits for the revealing of the sons of God."[24] Christ is the greatest teacher, and only He has the supremacy and generosity to make you great without adding any sorrow to your greatness. In fact, His job description on the cross of Calvary was the ultimate price He paid for the salvation of your soul, and only the greatest can pay such a heavy price for your redemption. Through Him, your success and greatness in life are guaranteed.

> *Success is not a function of where you work;*
> *it is a function of self-discovery and gift development.*

Do you want real-time and everlasting success? Then develop your God-given talent. You are the salt of the world, and the salt in you is your gift. You can preserve and beautify the world by developing your gift. The reward of developing your gift makes you a shining light on a mountaintop, radiating your glory for all to see. When you develop your gift, no one can stop your success; no matter how long it takes, you will manifest. Stand up, wake up, and pursue great things, because greatness is your birthright. Everything is possible.

> *You are a seed of Abraham; greatness is your birthright.*

The benefits of wisdom

His Word speaks to us: "My child, don't lose sight of good planning and insight. Hang on to them, for they fill you with life and bring you honor and respect. They keep you safe on your way [to greatness] and keep your feet from stumbling."[25]

> *What, then, is wisdom?*

> *Wisdom makes everything possible.*

Wisdom is not just the ability to apply knowledge, but it is also the strength that compels you to act on the knowledge you have acquired. If I have the ability to write this book but did not write it, that would mean I was not wise. However, wisdom has compelled me to write it. Having the ability is not good enough; acting on the ability does better.

The wisdom of God has the command to oblige you to do what should be done. Wisdom is not dormant; it is noticeable by action.

Wisdom is insight into reality and foresight into the future. Wisdom enables you to understand what ordinary people cannot see or understand. Wisdom or money can get you almost anything, but it's important to know that only wisdom can save your life. Money can buy only what you can see; therefore, money cannot save your life from HIV/AIDS, which has no cure for now. Wisdom alone can save your life from an unseen tragedy like HIV/AIDS and other earthly mishaps. Money cannot buy or produce wisdom, but wisdom produces treasure supernaturally, beyond the greatest abundance.

The following explanation of wisdom is from Proverbs 2 (NLT):

My child, listen to me and treasure my instructions.

Tune your ears to wisdom, and concentrate on understanding.

Cry out for insight and understanding.

Search for them as you would for lost money or hidden treasure

Then you will understand what it means to fear the Lord, and you will gain knowledge of God.

For the LORD grants wisdom! From his mouth come knowledge and understanding.

He grants a treasure of good sense to the godly.

He is their shield, protecting those who walk with integrity.

He guards the paths of justice and protects those who are faithful to him.

Then you will understand what is right, just and fair, and you will know how to find the right course of action every time.

For wisdom will enter your heart, and knowledge will fill you with joy.

Wise planning will watch over you. Understanding will keep you safe.

Wisdom will save you from evil people, from those whose speech is corrupt.

These people turn from right ways to walk down dark and evil paths.

They rejoice in doing wrong, and they enjoy evil as it turns things upside down.

What they do is crooked, and their ways are wrong.

Wisdom will save you from the immoral woman, from the flattery of the adulterous woman.

She has abandoned her husband and ignores the covenant she made before God.

Entering her house leads to death; it is the road to hell.

The man who visits her is doomed. He will never reach the paths of life.

Follow the steps of good men instead, and stay on the paths of the righteous.

For only the upright will live in the land, and those who have integrity will remain in it.

But the wicked will be removed from the land, and the unfaithful will be destroyed.

It is amazing to know that only wisdom can *save you from an immoral woman and from the flattery of the adulterous woman.* Immorality begets AIDS, and wisdom will save your life from immorality. So . . .

. . . Happy is the person who finds wisdom and gains understanding. For the profit of wisdom is better than silver, and her wages are better than gold. . . . Nothing you desire can compare with her. . . . She offers you long life in her right hand, and riches and honor in her left . . . Wisdom is a tree of life to those who embrace her; happy are those who hold her tightly. . . .

By wisdom, the LORD founded the earth; by understanding he established the heavens. By his knowledge, the deep fountains of the earth burst forth, and the clouds poured down rain.[26]

Wisdom is the means to attaining the best of every end.

Wisdom is what compels you to act excellently, exceptionally, and outstandingly under all circumstances, even under intense pressure. With wisdom, your judgment will be more accurate than you ever thought it could be. Wisdom is the means to attaining the best of every end. Wisdom is the most important thing—therefore, get wisdom!

Where can wisdom be found?

The Scripture says Man does not know its value [Wisdom], nor is it found in the land of the living but also the Scripture says again that:

"In him [Christ] lie hidden all the treasures of wisdom and knowledge." [27]

It is amazing to know that wisdom and excellence of knowledge are not located in any region of the world but are in Christ, and Christ is everywhere. The key to access wisdom and knowledge remains hidden in Christ until you receive, believe, and follow Christ. Until then, it will not be delivered to you. As soon as Christ dwells in you, wisdom and knowledge are automatically revealed unto you, giving you an uncompromised supernatural access to the wisdom that created this world and enabling you to function in the capacity of an undefeatable champion. Christ is the mighty power of God and the wonderful wisdom of God. Let the Word of God be the guarding principle in your life, and it will produce wisdom such that your life will count for riches, honor, greatness, and eternity. Christ is the Mount Zion, and the joy of the whole earth is Mount Zion. Champions do not belong to the base of the mountain, but they belong to the top of the mountain, where they can never be defeated again. Champions must grow in grace, meditation, and knowledge of Christ.

Reading God's Word without meditation is labor lost.

Reading and meditating on the Word of God is what produces divine knowledge, wisdom, and understanding. Within these three attributes is the fuel that will take you to the top of the mountain, and at the mountaintop, your life will produce such a wonderful success that no one will be able to gainsay it. Reach out for the Word, go for it and meditate on it and act in accordance with all that is written in it. You belong to the mountaintop. You are a champion; start living like one. You were born to operate from the mountaintop; don't sit at its base, and don't hang from its middle. Go for more knowledge of Christ and be on the mountaintop forever. "Everything is possible."

Champions see beyond life's obstacles
and failures because they are always on top.

Assurance for achieving greatness in life

We have been given knowledge about how to *ask* and *think*. Here is the unalterable assurance we have from God to buttress our faith, according to the Scripture: "Now unto Him [God] that is able to do exceeding abundantly above all that we ask or think, according to the power that worketh in us."[28]

This is eternal assurance that God is omnipotent; therefore, He is more than able to do all things. Our thoughts can reach a wider range than our prayer, but the Scripture assures us that God is able to do for us exceedingly beyond both our prayer requests and our hearts' desires. *This Scripture establishes the assertion that both our prayers and our thoughts have equal access to God, and the combination of the two will enable us to fly above and beyond the highest altitude that an airplane or jet ever flew.* We ask in prayer, and we generate thought by meditating on God's Word, so meditation is the act of using our minds to imagine possibilities and to break through every barrier and limitation, far beyond the limits of our physical ability. Powerful ideas are equally generated by meditation, because it is in meditation that we receive revelation, and revelation, if worked upon, can produce the desired manifestation.

You can gather your thoughts, but the Lord gives the right answer. Stand up with boldness in your heart and meditate on God's Word daily until God manifests the fulfillment of your dreams and visions. You have the assurance, the talent, the gift, and the capacity to receive from God. You need to wake up and claim the ends of the earth for your possession by being diligent at realizing your dream. This is your statutory right as a child of God. Come out of the darkness and let the world see your light shining. You are recognized as a child of the light, and light is the only thing that can overshadow darkness. No matter the darkness, it is not enough to put out the light in you. In other words, absolutely nothing is strong enough to stop your manifestation. Just take the step of faith and launch into the deep, because there are blessings in the deep. The Scripture says, ". . . the Almighty who blesses you with blessings of heaven above, blessings of the deep that lies beneath."[29] The blessings of heaven shall be on your head. Just launch out into the deep and allow the light of God in you to shine. Take action now; if you do not, your dream will remain only a pipe dream. Giants cannot kill a dream; what kills a dream is the fear of the giants, and to overcome the fear of the giants, move toward the giants and dislodge them by taking uncompromised actions. You are assured of the best covenant of *manifestation*; you will not be disappointed nor be put to shame.

I always rejoice that God is on the throne of grace, dispensing His mercy day and night. Do not deny yourself this blank check opportunity. Approach the throne of our gracious God with full confidence in your heart, and you will receive mercy and find grace to help you in time of need. Yes, there are many uncertainties in the world today. Government policies can change, climate might change, global warming could threaten humanity, resources might be scarce, the sea may overflow its boundaries, immigration laws may change, gas prices might keep increasing, the stock market might fluctuate, and companies might be cutting jobs as a result of the economic meltdown. But one thing is certain: the Word of God. If you stick to it and live by it, you will come out with testimonies of *manifestation.*

This is the voice of the Almighty God again saying to you right now, "You are my son. Today I have become your father. Only ask, and I will give you the nations as your inheritance, the ends of the earth as your possession."[30] What a stunning treaty! But here is what the Scripture says about fulfilling your side of the treaty: "If you stay joined to me [Christ] and my words remain in you, you may ask any request you like, and it will be granted!"[31] This is a blank check, and *if* you meet this condition, I am sure that your joy will overflow every earthly limit.

The earnest expectation of the creation eagerly awaits the manifestation of the sons of God.

CHAPTER THIRTEEN
POVERTY, CORRUPTION, AND AIDS

What is poverty?

In general, poverty is regarded as hunger, lack of shelter, uncertainty about the future, not having access to clean water, living in a polluted environment, lack of hope, lack of material wealth, lack of money, and lack of power. Every aspect of underdevelopment in the economy is regarded as poverty. As an economist, I learned to define poverty as above, but the question that has remained unanswered is that if anyone is hungry or sick and another gives him food or heals him, does that mean he is no longer poor?

This definition has created a wrong mindset about poverty and led many in a wrong direction. I once thought like this, as well, until I invited Christ into my vessel and read the Scripture that says, "Do not be conformed to this world, but be transformed by the renewing of your mind."[1] This powerful Scripture means that you must not subject yourself to any earthly principles or definition but must renew your mind with heavenly principles and definitions. This Scripture gives me a new mindset, and now I can say that poverty is more about ignorance than any other lack. Lack of material wealth does not make us poor, and acquisition of material wealth does not make us rich. Even if you have all the money in the whole world, if your mind still tells you that you are poor, then you are indeed a poor person. Your thinking makes you judge whether you are poor or rich.

"For one's life does not consist in the abundance of the things he possesses."[2]

Some say that poverty is not having a job. No, this thinking is too conventional. You are not poor because you are jobless; you are poor because you are ignorant of the powerful Scripture that says, "Out of his [your] heart shall flow rivers of living water."[3] In other words, within you is a great potential to be a job creator I am saying that you can move the cloud and shape the world to your state. Do not focus on being offered a job because you are well qualified or because you graduated from one of the best academic institutions; instead, focus on your capacity and potential to manifest as a child of God.

Your degree merely prepares you for the life assignment that God has placed you on earth to fulfill. For instance, my educational background as an economist with a national diploma in computer science made fulfilling the assignment of writing this book much easier and more realistic. God sees my qualifications as a prerequisite to fulfilling His assignment for my life. The idea seemed extremely difficult, but believe me, everything is possible with God. Look within yourself now and you will hear a song that says *you can do everything through Christ who strengthens you.*[4] It is the strength of Christ in you that makes accomplishing your dream possible. To go that extra mile in life and become an outstanding person, you must totally depend on Christ's strength.

The world's definition of poverty has generated inordinate desires in the hearts of many people, making them want more and more material things. And such a disposition of mind is never fulfilled. In fact, acquiring HIV/AIDS is one of the consequences of such a disposition of mind. Some have used the sex trade as a channel for meeting more of their basic needs. Today, poverty seems to be the underpinning of the sex trade, and there is a high prevalence of HIV/AIDS among people

who practice the sex trade. Why? Because people are *ignorant* of what the Scripture says, which is *that your life does not consist in the abundance of the materials things you possess.* In other words, comfort, wisdom, happiness, honor, and riches do not depend on how much money you have or the abundance of material goods you possess. Rather, they depend on God, who is the author and preserver of your life. That is why Scripture tells us that "when the poor and needy seek water, and there is none, and their tongue faileth for thirst, I, the Lord will hear them, I the God of Israel will not forsake them."[5]

The inordinate desire for money and material goods has induced many, especially young people and college students, to engage in the sex trade. Today, many are living with HIV, and many more are on the verge of entering that same ugly trade. This is not really because of poverty; it is due more to a high level of ignorance, the same kind of ignorance that led the people of ancient times into sexual immorality, causing thousands of them to die. I deeply believe that the socioeconomic problems associated with poverty, including lack of access to high-quality health care, can directly or indirectly increase the risk of HIV infection. Young people who have dropped out of school are more likely to become sexually active and to engage in the sex trade. They want to make a living, irrespective of the nature of the job. This notion is totally wrong, because you do not make a living by using your body; you make a living by using your potential.

Once having seen through this misconception, adolescents need accurate, age-appropriate information about HIV/AIDS infection. They also need to learn how to talk with their parents or other trusted adults about HIV/AIDS, how to reduce or eliminate risk factors, how to talk with a potential partner about risk factors, and where to get tested for HIV/AIDS. Their minds must be renewed and reprogrammed. They must understand Godly standards and follow them. This responsibility rests on the shoulders of the parents, so *start nurturing your children at home at an early stage of life. Only an embryo that is well nurtured will eventually become a toddler.*

"Let there be no sexual immorality, impurity or greed among you. Such sins have no place among God's people." [6]

Poverty reduces self-esteem. Our lives are too precious to be traded for sex or sold for billions of dollars. Do not trade your future for ruin.

Never take part in worthless, evil, and dark deeds; instead, rebuke and expose them. Come out boldly to speak against your friends who engage in the sex trade; speak against teachers who ask for sex in return for a passing grade; speak against human resources personnel who ask for sex in return for employment; speak against a manager or boss who asks you for sex in return for a promotion; speak against any politician who uses his or her political position to lure you into sex. In addition to being corrupt, some of these people may be HIV-positive.

The pleasure you derive from engaging in an unholy sex might be considerable, but the consequences are catastrophic and could put your life in jeopardy. *What is pleasurable today may be a source of pain tomorrow.*

Having little or no money need not translate into low self-esteem. The quality of your life is inestimable; it is worth more than billions of dollars, so do not be deceived into casual sex for gain, because it will ruin your future. Do not be deceived into the sex trade. It is horrible: it leads to prostitution, and it shows a lack of self-discipline. Prostitution is a bottomless pit. If you engage in it, you will groan in anguish when disease consumes your body; you will come to the brink of utter ruin; and you will definitely face public disgrace when diseases like HIV blossom in your body. The result of casual sex is as bitter as poison and as sharp as a double-edged sword.

A word is enough for the wise. Run away from the sex trade, irrespective of your economic situation or how deep you have sunk into it. Just believe the Word of God that says, "Even strong young lions sometimes go hungry, but those who trust in the Lord will never lack any good thing."[7] Submit your case to God; present your arguments to Him, and He will turn your desert into a pool of water. Only God, our Redeemer, the Holy One of Israel, can bring water out of the rock. Please seek God. With God, "everything is possible." Yes, it is.

"The lazy man does not roast what he took in hunting, but diligence is man's precious possession."[8]

Permit me to share this great testimony with you. Just after I finished my national service assignment, I was without a job. Things were not looking too good, but this Scripture came alive to me: "Those who look to him [God] for help will be radiant with joy; no shadow of shame will darken their faces."⁹ I committed myself to Him, and I was diligently searching for what to do. In a short time, this scripture manifested in my life, and business opportunities began to show up. This was the scripture that liberated me from the fear of poverty. Believe me, with God's revelation there is always a way to bring water out of the rock. All it takes is diligence and perseverance. With or without a job, do not ever remain idle. Keep working toward your dream, because the hand of diligence will make you rich. Prophecy tells us that a diligent man has the grace to stand before kings and sit with the elites.¹⁰ Today, I will continue to thank God for where I am and for preserving my personal seat among the elites. We must no longer believe the skeptics, but believe in the supremacy of the word that says "everything is possible."

"For this reason, I also suffer these things;
nevertheless I am not ashamed,
for I know whom I have believed and am persuaded that He is
able to keep what I have committed to Him until that Day."¹¹

You too have a reserved seat among the elites; you equally possess the tools to get everything done. Your presence anywhere warrants a standing ovation, but please be diligent at pursuing your dream and vision. As I am writing now, I can sense God is saying to someone that He is your shepherd and that He has given you everything you need to make a blissful journey on this earth. God is also telling you not to doubt Him, but only to believe that you are who God says you are. God is saying that He created you to multiply and subdue the earth. God has put you in charge of everything He made, giving you authority over all things. It is amazing to know that all the money in the world cannot buy a dot of what God can do in your life.

It is time for us to speak out and tell young people who engage in casual sex to stop regarding sex as a leisure activity or a business transaction. Do not regard your body as a medium of exchange for goods or services. This notion is completely wrong. Your future will be doomed because of such acts. Your life is about more than money or whatever other purpose that exists behind your reason for casual sex or prostitution. God made you a fruitful and productive creature. You are fearfully and wonderfully made. Make things happen for yourself. The power to succeed is in you. Channel this power to pursue excellent things, and the reward will be extraordinary. According to Scripture, wealth made through prostitution or the sex trade is an "ill-gotten gain [that] brings no lasting happiness; right living does."[12]

No degree of poverty justifies engaging in the sex trade or prostitution.

There is nothing that is worth more than the soul. Do not joke with the issues of HIV/AIDS; it is real and very common. Do not become a victim before you have to believe that AIDS IS REAL. The sex trade is a road that leads to an early grave. Stay off this road. Watch your back very well; otherwise you might not survive your next act of sex. I reject this for your life, and my prayer is that God will renew your mind so that you can start living a life that glorifies His name. Throw off your old evil nature and your former way of life, which was full of lust and deception and rotten through and through. Let there be a spiritual renewal of your thoughts and attitudes. It does not matter how your past has been. God does not look at your past to bless you, because He knows you are a precious gem in His kingdom. You will not perish by His grace. You must display a new nature that is in Christ, because you are now a new person created in God's likeness, which is righteous, holy, and true. Only true repentance and asking God for forgiveness through his Son can bring about a renewal of your mind and change in your thinking. Lack of material wealth does not make you a poor being. The desire to acquire more material things is based on the misconception that happiness comes from getting more, but this is not true at all. It will provide only momentary joy. Your identity worth is greater than your disposable worth; your value is not and can never be determined by your valuables.

How to conquer poverty

Poverty can be conquered by conquering your thoughts. God gave you the ability to imagine; He gave you creative imagination. You are meant to use your power of imagination to focus on the abundant resources God has put at your disposal. When you dwell on what you do not have, your negative feelings will make you begin to think that you are poor. No, lacking material things does not make you poor; what makes you poor is your negative thinking pattern. Spend more time dwelling on God's Word, which promises you abundance and victory in life through Jesus Christ. God dwells in you, and the Scripture says of Christ, "Worthy is the Lamb who was slain to receive power, and riches, and wisdom, and strength, and honor, and glory, and blessings!"[13]

These seven ingredients were packaged for you before the foundation of the earth was laid, so start seeing yourself as a prosperous person with unending riches and honor. Begin to see yourself reaching the mountaintop of the highest position in life without compromising your good values. Begin to see yourself creating a business that will flourish like a tree planted along the riverbank, which never fails to bear fruit in every season.[14] Even when your present situation has not changed, just believe in your God and dream big. Start seeing yourself living with abundant resources. Believe that God created you to be a winner, not a loser. He gave you the supernatural capacity to succeed, irrespective of your past or your background. God is the source of your life. Focus on His Word, and the whole world will celebrate your success. Poverty is not your destiny. Remember, there is an end, but the expectations of a child of God must come to manifestation.

Poverty is never your destiny.

Poverty is a mindset that focuses on lack of material acquisition of wealth as a yardstick for measuring success. Poverty is a wrong mindset.

"As a man thinks in his heart, so is he."[15] If you can change the way you think, you can change the way you live, as well. Your outer is the actual product of your inner. Your way of thinking must change completely. By that I mean that your mind has to be repositioned to think more positively and correctly. You must have a *possibility mentality*. You must absolutely believe that you can change your world by thinking more positively and having a positive mental picture of what you intend to become. This kind of right thinking gives way to the realization of mighty visions, dreams, and opportunities. Martin Luther King Jr. thought in this manner years ago, and today the world has certainly manifested his positive mentality.

Shapeless destiny can be shaped by a positive mentality.

Our past heroes were great and committed thinkers who made a huge impact in their time just by thinking in terms of "possibilities" at all times. If you can change your thinking, you can change your life. A negative thinking pattern can lead you into reckless behavior. Your mentality can shape your destiny.

Personally, I see what I do not have as what I do not need, because if I need or want something, my God will provide it. The Scripture says, "My God shall supply all your need according to His riches in glory by Christ Jesus."[16] This unchangeable principle is what I meditate on day and night. Today, this principle has changed my own personal perspective about poverty, and I give God the glory because of His signature on my life and affairs. Christ said He has wiped out the handwriting of ordinances against me, which was contrary to me, and took it out of my way, nailing it to His cross and replacing it with His signature.[17] Christ did it for all creatures, and all who also believe and live by this standard today live in abundance.

Now you have the choice to live by this principle so that you too can live in abundance. You have the choice to think positively, to focus more on what you have than on what you do not have. Your choice is you. Poverty is a function of ignorance or lack of understanding. I am sure a good understanding can take us completely out of poverty, and lack of it can create hardship. Remember always, "Trust in the LORD with all your heart, and do not rely on your own understanding; think about Him in all your ways, and He will guide you on the right paths."[18]. All the tools to succeed are ready-made and available; the only problem is our mindset. You can conquer poverty; you can have success beyond measure because everything is possible.

Understanding corruption and HIV/AIDS

A world without corruption is possible.
"Everything is possible."

What is corruption?

Corruption occurs when organizations or individuals profit improperly from their position in the world and their activities. Corruption can be found in all countries but is more common in countries with weak and undeveloped legal, communication, and public administration systems.

Corruption can hold back the efficiency of the HIV/AIDS awareness campaign, as well as prevention and treatment, if earmarks for public education and treatments are misappropriated or diverted for personal use by corrupt personnel. The comparatively expensive nature of HIV/AIDS antiretroviral drugs makes them vulnerable to corrupt diversion; counterfeit drugs can be made to replace genuine drugs. Money can be made from the resale of HIV/AIDS drugs that were originally supplied at preferential prices to poor countries. Healthcare officials can request illicit payments for treatment or service delivery that was meant to be free. Donations from the international community, foundations, NGOS, and private organizations are meant to assist poor countries so they can deliver HIV/AIDS treatments free, but the activities of corrupt officials can impede reaching the number of people who are meant to get these treatments or the public education they need, which may frustrate donor countries or organizations. *My prayer is that God will frustrate every device of these crafty operations that seek to impede developmental goals and objectives so that their hands cannot carry out their plans.*

Fighting corruption should become the most important policy we need to pursue, and we should do so with both physical and spiritual strength. Corrupt citizens are determined to ruin nations, to give nations a bad reputation locally and internationally, to destroy the economy, to undermine democracy, and to destroy the future of our youth. Upright citizens must also be well determined to make sure that the rule of law is well followed and justice is well applied to every corrupt citizen, irrespective of his or her political position or economic power. Corruption does not benefit nations; rather, some criminally minded personalities see corruption as the way to make ill-gotten gains.

Corruption:

- Causes poverty
- Destroys economies
- Gives countries a bad image
- Leads to poor service delivery
- Denies social amenities to the people
- Frustrates indigenous professionalism, innovation, creativity, hard work, and entrepreneurship
- Causes the collapse of local industries
- Destroys the future of our youth
- Undermines democracy
- Impacts human rights severely
- Weakens the rules of law

Corruption is not a direct cause of HIV/AIDS, but corruption seriously weighs down the effectiveness of the HIV/AIDS awareness campaign, prevention, and treatment. The social cost of corruption is enormous and should be at all times prevented by solid policies that make corruption absolutely impossible. Let's say no to corruption.

Public and private office holders have the mandatory duty to manage the resources entrusted to them. Honesty and accountability should be the watchwords. No one is above the law. Remember, one day you will be accountable to God.

CHAPTER FOURTEEN
WORD OF KNOWLEDGE:
CAN GOD CALL YOU A MAN?

My people are destroyed for lack of knowledge. Because you have rejected knowledge, I also will reject you from being priest for Me. Because you have forgotten the law of your God, I also will forget your children.[1]

The Bible defines a man as someone who teaches his household and his neighbors in the way of the Lord. No matter how influential you are, if your character falls short of this kingdom principle, *you are not a man*. A man is not defined by the qualities he has that enable him to perform certain functions, but by his virtues and character. Money, position, title, and fame do not buy character. Money, position, title, and fame are good things, but without character they are meaningless. When God looked down on Sodom and Gomorrah, He said, "I sought for a man among them who would make a wall, and stand in the gap before Me on behalf of the land, that I should not destroy it; but I found no one."[2] Remember, Mr. Lot was the equivalent of a billionaire, and his two potential sons-in-law were also there, but God did not recognize them as men because they came short of the qualities God expects in a man. A man diffuses kingdom principles to his household and the others around him, and God intervenes.

Do not end up in a cave as Lot did. Our end should be more glorious than our beginning. Abraham, our father, had a splendid life from the beginning to the end, and he died at a good old age. You are the result of this covenant but can come short of it through acts of greediness, selfishness, self-centeredness, ignorance, covetousness, hostility, disobedience, and lack of moral values.

I want you to work on this consciousness, that no matter what world reports say about low life expectancy, you will become an old man full of years, like your father Abraham. Have you not heard that he that is from above is above all? You are above life challenges and disease. Every earthly report is based on current circumstances, which are subject to change, whereas the Word is changeless, and faith in the Word was empowered by the blood of Jesus before the earth was ever created. Sit down with the Word of God and learn the principles an overcomer needs to overcome all life situations and challenges.

Men, as the head of your families, you are the Abraham of your family. Right now, establish core moral standards of sincerity, truth, integrity, honesty, and hard work. These values are the best inheritance you can give your children; these values are better and more important than heaps of money; they are real, money-producing values; they are the values that will give your family, in scriptural terms, the ability to "dominate and subdue," by which I am referring to dominion and command.

Family values must be built on core moral standards so that we can protect members of our immediate families and society at large. It bothers the heart of God so much when core moral standards are not established, and He depends on you as the head of the family to command your household in the way of the Lord. Do not be discouraged. It might seem difficult, but with the help of God, everything is possible. Second Chronicles 15:7 (NLT) says "For your work shall be rewarded, says the LORD." You will not perish, you will not lose your possessions, and you will not end your life in a cave. There is hope in the future of your family; your children shall come back to their own border. It is absolutely possible for your family to live a life of moral excellence and supernatural success and for you to live without AIDS.

God added so much value to our lives by giving us the Holy Spirit. The Scripture says we are made in God's image. It is crucial for every creation of God to add value to others' lives. This is the path to greatness. A little input from you can turn the life of another around for the better. Let's give back to the society in which we belong. This is what the good news of Christ is all about, and this is also the best way to take the good news around the world. Good is what overcomes evil. By continuing to do good, you will overcome evil in the name of Jesus.

As you establish core moral standards at the heart of your family and as you take steps to teach your household the way of the Lord, in accordance with and obedient to God's Word, the blessing of God will supernaturally locate you and manifest. "And you shall know the truth, and the truth shall make you free."[3] The Scripture tells us, "Sanctify them by Your truth. Your word is truth."[4] It also says, ". . . for You [God] has magnified Your [His] word above Your [His] name."[5] The Word of God is the principle of God. Sanctify your family today with kingdom principles, and they will reflect the very best and true nature of God.

Do you want to be counted as a man? Begin diffusing kingdom principles, first to your family, and then taking the step of faith to other families around you. This is how to claim nations as your inheritance--by taking gradual steps of faith. You are on your way to greatness. God's divine power has given you everything that pertains to life and Godliness, so to you *everything is possible.* Yes, it is possible.

Understand that I have already given a clue about Lot's and Eli's families and how their families ended, and I think it will do us good to end with the family of the greatest man of all the people of the East. His name was Job. He was a blameless and an upright man. God made a hedge around his household and his properties on every side. God blessed the work of his hands, and his possessions increased in the land. God did all these things for Job because he was righteous and had a regular custom of sanctifying his children by rising up early in the morning to pray for them all. Job went through difficult times, but his end was overwhelming peace. According to the Scriptures, "Mark the blameless man, and observe the upright; for the future of that man is peace."[6] The end of Job's family justifies the fulfillment of this Scripture.

If all parents can learn from Job's family and sanctify their children with the truth, God will build a hedge around their households and their properties on every side. Yes, God will bless the work of your hands, and your possessions will increase in the land. It will not matter what challenges are facing your family now, because, believe me, the future of your family shall be overwhelming peace because the Scripture tells us that "the Strength of Israel will not lie nor relent. For He is not a man that He should relent."[7]

What makes everything possible is not what we see or hear but what we believe. Seeing and hearing alone do not themselves attract grace, but belief based on the supremacy of the Word of God has no comparison. You might have seen the impossible become possible; you might have heard that everything is possible, but to him who believes, everything *is* possible. Yes, it is.

The immorality that was found in Sodom and Gomorrah is also available in the twenty-first century. Today, there might not be cities like Sodom and Gomorrah were in the ancient times, yet today, some families represent Sodom and Gomorrah and are on the brink of being destroyed by *HIV/AIDS,* or *WASTING DISEASE.* This book can be a significant gift to such a family. Someone who is reading this book right now needs to keep in touch with God by sending this book or other eye-opening and valuable materials to liberate such families from the ignorance that seems to be the greatest enemy of mankind. The Scripture says "Therefore my people have gone into captivity, because they have no knowledge."[8] Knowledge can sets such family free from ignorance.

Lot, who lived in a mansion in the city of Sodom, failed to spread the knowledge of God he had learned from his uncle, Abraham. He failed to share or give to others, and he died sickly in a cave. God took away the discretion, audacity, and the swiftness that had made him a father, and he lost all he had through his sluggishness. The simple act of sharing and giving can increase the discretion, audacity, and swiftness that would qualify us for high placement in life.

A man who has riches without understanding is like the beasts that perish

This simple act of providing the gift of valuable information can give other families the chance to live out their dreams; it can save and transform many lives. The greatest joy comes when you share what you know with others and give to others imperishable and valuable gifts. *It takes joy to draw water from the wells of salvation.* Do not behave as if the problems of society do not concern you. No matter how well-placed your mansion is, *if you refuse to influence your society and claim nations as your inheritance, the society will forcefully influence you and claim you as its inheritance.* This is what happened to Lot. He lacked understanding, the society influenced him and he became like the Sodomites. God will not be disappointed when you manifest as a billionaire, because that has been His perfect will for you, even before you were born. However, God *will be* disappointed if you refuse to claim nations as your inheritance. Stay in touch with God by sharing your knowledge with others and giving them what is beneficial. The Bible says that we should, above all, keep our love for one another at full strength, because *LOVE COVERS A MULTITUDE OF SINS.*[9]

Please pray this prayer right now!

> *I confess my impotence and weakness to my Lord. Have mercy upon me, O God. Forgive my past sluggishness and create in me a clean heart and renew a steadfast spirit within me. Do not cast me away from Your presence, and do not take Your Holy Spirit from me. Restore to me the joy of Your salvation and uphold me by Your generous Spirit. Spirit of Liberty, empower me to teach my household and my neighbors Your kingdom principles and make me your vessel to influence and convert many to Your kingdom of light. In the name of Jesus. Amen.*

This is the empowerment that you need to succeed as a father; this is the banner of strength that you need to receive nations as your inheritance. Whenever you sincerely confess your impotence or incompetence, you will have undeniable access to Omnipotence. That is why the Scripture says, "Not that we are sufficient of ourselves to think of anything as being from ourselves, but our sufficiency is from God."[10] The Scripture says, "In the same way, Sodom and Gomorrah and the cities around them committed sexual immorality and practiced perversions, just as they did, and serve as an example by undergoing the punishment of eternal fire."[11]

"In His days the righteous shall flourish, and abundance of peace, until the moon is no more" [1]

Use Mr. Lot as a case study, and conclude right now to be a different father with a different spirit full of understanding. Remember in the word of the Scripture that Caleb the son of Jephunneh, the Kenizzit was saved and not destroyed with the rest because God said he had a different spirit in him and had followed God fully.[13] Place your faith in God. *Faith is conclusion without evidence.* Your conclusion about Christ is your total belief in the supremacy of His words, and Christ will manifest Himself in your conclusion. The world needs your input; do not die the way Lot died, because nothing of great significance could be said about him. Today, decide to have a different spirit like Caleb did and your household shall manifest greatness. Join the race to stop AIDS, uphold morality at all levels, and believe that together we can exterminate AIDS. This is my conclusion because, with God, "everything is possible."

CHAPTER FIFTEEN
DESTROYING THE YOKE OF HIV
THROUGH PRAYER

With God, everything is possible.[1]

At the hour of prayer, which was the ninth hour, Peter spoke to the lame man at the gate, calling out the beautiful words, "In the name of Jesus Christ of Nazareth, rise up and walk."[2] He lifted him up, and immediately, his feet and bones received strength—and the man walked.

It is your time and hour to receive the strength to overcome what the doctors have considered impossible. Doctors are human beings. What seems impossible to human beings is possible with God. Don't consider your doctor's report as final; consider the Word of God as having final authority over your life.

The Scripture says, "In those days was Hezekiah sick unto death. And the prophet Isaiah, the son of Amoz came to him, and said unto him, Thus saith the Lord, Set thine house in order; for thou shalt die, and not live."[3] The conclusion to be made here is that Hezekiah had an incurable disease and received a report that, in our time, would be referred to as a doctor's report. This report came directly from God, and Hezekiah wondered what could reverse this divine pronouncement.

So Hezekiah prayed unto the Lord (See 2 Kings 20:2-6), and God condescended to grant his request. God answered Hezekiah's prayer and sent the same prophet, Isaiah, to tell Hezekiah that God had added more years to his life. The greatness of God and the power of prayer changed Hezekiah's impossible situation.

Brothers and sisters, nothing is impossible to prayer, because absolutely nothing is impossible to the ever-winning God. There are things in life that human beings and science cannot revoke, but you can experience the wonders of God through prayer. God can change the situation. With God, everything is possible.

Have you received a report that tells you, in effect, to go home and wait to die? Are you crying as Hezekiah did? Do not weep again. Behold, the Lion of the tribe of Judah, the Root of David, has prevailed over your disease. Christ was sent to die for *you*, and He did this with His precious blood, which is without blemish. It pleased the Lord to bruise Him and put Him to grief. God afflicted Him with your sicknesses,[4] which means that Christ was afflicted with HIV/AIDS and cancer. The body of Christ had the capacity to absorb what your body cannot absorb. All forms of diseases were nailed with Him to the cross. His body was able to bear that great burden. Sickness belongs to the cross, not to your body; so stand up now and start commanding that disease to go back to the cross. This is what it means to cast your burden upon Him.

Go back to the cross!

Let us call forth a new slogan: *"Go back to the cross!"* As the Scripture says, "Cast your burden on the Lord, and He shall sustain you; He shall never permit the righteous to be moved."[5] All forms of sickness are a burden, and sickness shall not have dominion over you. Do not weep again. Behold, the Lion of the tribe of Judah, the Root of David, has prevailed over your disease. Christ took our infirmities and bore our diseases, and He gave us all authority to be master over demons and diseases. It has been fulfilled. You are the master over every circumstance that has placed you in bondage. Don't cry. Don't weep. Just *speak*, and *command* sickness to *go back to the cross*, using the precious name of Jesus. Take your stand now. God will heed your voice as He heeded the voice of Hezekiah in his affliction.

Remember, God will do as you have spoken to His hearing. *What you speak determines what you get.*

At the ninth hour, the name of Jesus Christ of Nazareth reversed the hopeless situation at the beautiful gate, and the lame man walked. This is your ninth hour, which is the hour of prayer. Keep speaking; don't stop commanding. The more you speak, the more you command, the more your voice will prevail over every circumstance, in the precious name of Jesus. Amen.

"Whoever calls on the name of the LORD shall be saved."[6]

Prayer for this hour

"Call upon Me in the day of trouble;
I will deliver you, and you shall glorify Me."[7]

Take every situation that looks hopeless to God, using the name of Jesus. Ask God to be merciful toward you and everything surrounding your life. Right now, regularly partake of the communion with the bread and the blood. Praise God and commit your situation into His able hands. "Whoever offers praise, glorifies Me; / And to him who orders his conduct aright, / I will show the salvation of God."[8] Today, The Sun of Righteousness shall arise for you with healing in His wings in name of Jesus. Remember, happy are the people whose God is the LORD![9]

"For this reason I also suffer these things;
nevertheless I am not ashamed,
for I know whom I have believed and am persuaded that He is
able to keep what I have committed to Him until that Day."[10]

Father, I pray for all the readers. May the heavens declare God's righteousness over you now, and I decree that every irrevocable situation and judgment in your life will be revoked by Jehovah, in the name of Jesus. Thank you, Lord. You are God who heals all diseases. I believe your people are healed because the Strength of Israel will not lie.

Finally, brothers and sisters, "I commend you to God and to the word of His grace, which is able to build you up and give you an inheritance among all those who are sanctified."[11] This is my conclusion: With God, everything is possible.

CHAPTER SIXTEEN
QUESTIONS FOR
REFLECTION AND DISCUSSION

Questions

1. HIV is a virus that attacks and weakens which system?
   A. Digestive system

   B. Immune system

   C. Circulatory system

2. Only drug users and gay men need to worry about becoming infected with HIV.
   True

   False

3. It is easy to tell whether someone is infected with HIV.
   True

   False

4. Which body fluid cannot transmit HIV?
   A. Blood

   B. Semen

   C. Vaginal fluids

   D. Breast milk

   E. Saliva

5. A vaccine is available to protect people from HIV infection.
   True

   False

6. Globally, most women become infected with HIV through:
    A. Childbirth

    B. Blood transfusions

    C. Drug injections

    D. Reckless sex

7. Young people under 25 now account for at least half of all new HIV infections in the world.
    True

    False

8. There is no link between HIV and other sexually transmitted diseases (STDs).
    True

    False

9. All people infected with HIV are aware of their status.
    True

    False

10. You can find out your HIV status by asking for:
    A. An HIV test

    B. A general physical examination

    C. A gynecological examination

11. What is opportunistic infection?

12. What is the immune system?

13. Why is HIV/AIDS testing important?

14. HIV/AIDS testing is important for pregnant women.

    True

    False

15. State three benefits of moral education.

16. Do I need to take any special precautions at work, at home, or when visiting friends?

17. Do I need to talk about HIV/AIDS to my parents, my friends, my family members, and my colleagues at work?

18. What is the role of white blood cells?

19. Can our white blood cells fight HIV/AIDS and prevent it from attacking us?

20. Body tattooing, incision, circumcision, and shaving can spread HIV/AIDS.

   True

   False

21. HIV/AIDS can spread through:
   A. Handshaking

   B. Hugging

   C. Blood contact

22. An HIV/AIDS-positive mother can transmit HIV virus to her baby through breastfeeding?

   True

   False

23. HIV/AIDS awareness/prevention is the key to reducing the infection rate.

   True

   False

24. HIV/AIDS can attack only people in Africa.

   True

   False

25. Why are high STD rates relevant to HIV/AIDS risk?

26. Why is body tattooing a risk factor for HIV/AIDS?

27. Are young people at risk of HIV/AIDS?

28. State three ways to prevent AIDS.

29. When is World AIDS Day held?

30. What is wasting disease?

The answers are available on the next pages. How did you do?

Further suggestions for
enhancing your understanding of HIV/AIDS

Do personal research on why HIV/AIDS is a global epidemic.

Write about your personal perspective on HIV/AIDS.

Answers

1. B) The immune system. HIV, the virus that causes AIDS, attacks and weakens the immune system by targeting certain cells that defend the body against illness.

2. False. Anyone can become infected with HIV.

3. False. You cannot tell by looking at someone whether he or she is infected with HIV.

4. (E) Saliva. HIV can be found in certain body fluids, such as blood, semen, pre-ejaculation secretions, vaginal secretions, and breast milk. HIV is NOT spread through casual contact such as hugging or shaking hands, and cannot be spread through contact with sweat, tears, or saliva.

5. False. There is no vaccine or cure for AIDS. Treatments are available that can help people live longer and delay the onset of AIDS. But the side effects are serious, and drug-resistant strains of the virus can make even the best medications ineffective. Prevention is the best defense against HIV/AIDS.

6. (D) Reckless sex. Worldwide, half of all people living with HIV/AIDS are women, and the majority of them were infected through reckless sex.

7. True. Young adults and teens continue to be at risk for HIV infection. Most young people are infected through reckless sex.

8. False. People with STDs may be more likely to contract HIV. It is also easier for those with other STDs to transmit the virus.

9. False. Most people infected with HIV do not know their status and might be unknowingly spreading the virus.

10. (A) An HIV test. The only way to know for sure whether you are HIV-positive is to take an HIV test.

11. Opportunistic Infection is an illness caused by an organism that usually does not cause disease in a person with a normal immune system. People with advance HIV infection suffer opportunistic infection of the brain, lungs, eye and the likes.

12. Immune system is the complex function of the body that recognizes foreign agents or substances, neutralize them and recall the response later when confronted with the same challenge.

13. HIV/AIDS testing is the only way to know whether a person has HIV/AIDS.

14. True. With HIV/AIDS testing, infected mothers will know they should not breastfeed their babies.

15. Benefits of a moral education:

    A. Moral education teaches us how to behave decently and honorably.

    B. Moral education helps us to recognize right from wrong so that we can make quality decisions.

    C. Moral education gives us acceptable standards of behavior.

16. No. The only risk is through contact with blood, semen, or vaginal fluids. HIV cannot be spread through everyday contact at home, at work, in the street, or in a restaurant. It cannot be spread through casual contact, such as shaking hands, hugging, and kissing.

17. Yes. It is good to talk to others about HIV/AIDS, because the more you talk about it, the more you will understand its nature, and the more lives you will save.

18. White blood cells help to fight diseases that attack our bodies, but the HIV/AIDS virus is stronger than a white blood cell. That is why HIV/AIDS can attack and eventually kill the body if you do not protect yourself with thorough knowledge about AIDS.

19. No. The HIV/AIDS virus is stronger than the white blood cells. HIV/AIDS attacks and weakens the white blood cells.

20. True. Body tattoos, circumcision, and shaving with unsterilized blades or knives can spread HIV/AIDS.

21. (C) Only blood contact can spread HIV/AIDS.

22. True. This is called mother-to-baby transmission. An HIV/AIDS-positive mother can transmit the HIV virus to her baby through her breast milk.

23. True. HIV/AIDS awareness/prevention is the key to reducing the infection rate and ultimately defeating AIDS.

24. False. HIV/AIDS is a global epidemic. It spreads rapidly both within countries and across their borders. It affects people regardless of gender, geographical location, or sexual orientation. The whole world is now faced with a multitude of AIDS epidemics.

25. Because reckless sex that results in the transmission of an STD could also result in HIV/AIDS transmission.

26. HIV/AIDS is spread when the blood or body fluids of an infected person enter the body of another person, either through a break in the skin or through a mucous membrane. Tattooing punctures the skin and is therefore an easy way to spread HIV/AIDS.

27. Yes. Young people are most vulnerable, and they are at risk if they have reckless sex, share needles, or engage in other high-risk behaviors.

28. Ways to prevent HIV/AIDS.

    A. Do not share instruments, such as razor blades, needles, and syringes.

    B. Cover cuts and wounds with waterproof bandages or a piece of clean cloth.

    C. Do not have sex until you are married and then remain faithful to your partner. Both partners should get an HIV/AIDS test before marriage.

    D. Total abstinence from sex is the most effective prevention measure.

29. Every year, December 1ST is world AIDS day.

30. How did you define wasting disease? Good Luck. I wish you a life full of God's blessings and miraculous.

NOTES

Note and Prologue

[1] Taken from Mark 10:27 HCSB: "Looking at them, Jesus said, 'With men it is impossible, but not with God, because all things are possible with God.'"

[2] Business the ultimate Resource 2nd Edition Page 1334

[3] Proverbs 11:4 NLT

[4] Proverbs 11:11 NLT

CHAPTER ONE:
HISTORICAL ACCOUNT OF THE KILLER DISEASE

[1] Ecclesiastes 1:9 HCSB

[2] Hosea 4:6 HCSB

[3] Numbers 25:1 NKJV

[4] Numbers 25:2-3 NKJV

[5] Leviticus 26:14-16 NKJV

[6] Leviticus 26:21 NKJV

[7] Deuteronomy 28:59 NKJV

[8] 1 Kings 18:19 ff

[9] Leviticus19:28 HCSB

[10] Deuteronomy 14:1-2 HCSB

[11] Proverbs 6:25 HCSB

[12] Ecclesiastes 4:12

CHAPTER TWO:
THE ESSENCE OF BLOOD

[1] Leviticus 17:11 HCSB

[2] John 10:10 HCSB

[3] http://www.unaids.org

[4] Proverbs 9:17 NASB

CHAPTER FOUR:
FORMULA TO PREVENT HIV INFECTION

[1] Proverbs 6:24 NLT

[2] Proverbs 6:26

[3] Proverbs 6:33 NLT

[4] Luke 1:37 NLT

[5] Isaiah 14:27 TLB

[6] Mark 11:24 NLT

[7] James 5:15

Chapter Five:
Sex

[1] Genesis 1:23 KJV

[2] 1 Timothy 4:12 HCSB

Chapter Six:
Abstinence

[1] 2 Corinthians 6:7-7:1 NLT

[2] 2 Timothy 4:12 HCSB

[3] Proverbs 18:22 NLT

[4] Proverbs 12:4 NLT

[5] Ecclesiastes 3:1 NIV

[6] Based on Deuteronomy 28:1 and Exodus 23:25

[7] Job 36:11 NLT

[8] Hebrews 12:11 NLT

[9] Based on Proverbs 14:34

CHAPTER SEVEN:
PARENTAL ROLE IN THE FIGHT AGAINST AIDS

[1] Malachi 4:6 HCSB

[2] Hosea 4:6 NLT

[3] Baker's Evangelical Dictionary of Biblical Theology. Edited by Walter A. Elwell. © 1996 by Walter A. Elwell. Published by Baker Books, a division of Baker Book House Company, Grand Rapids, Michigan 49516-6287.

[4] Genesis 18:19 HCSB

[5] 2 Chronicles 28:19

[6] Proverbs 29:15

[7] Proverbs 22:6 TLB

[8] John 8:32

[9] John 17:17

[10] Psalm 138:2

[11] Proverbs 22:6

[12] Genesis 11:6

[13] 2 Timothy 1:5

[14] Matthew 19:14

CHAPTER EIGHT:
THE ROLE OF YOUTH IN PREVENTING AIDS

[1] Exodus 20:12

[2] Deuteronomy 6:6-7 HCSB

[3] Psalm 78:4 NLT

[4] Philippians 4:8

[5] Ayo Daniels (See Notes)

CHAPTER NINE:
HIV/AIDS, COURTSHIP, AND MARRIAGE

[1] Deuteronomy 7:14 NIV

[2] Isaiah 60:22 NLT

[3] Colossians 3:5 NLT

[4] Proverbs 12:2

[5] Philippians 4:13

[6] Ephesians 5:24 NLT

[7] 1 Peter 3:7 NLT

[8] Galatians 5:22

[9] 1 Corinthians 13:21

CHAPTER TEN:
THE CURE FOR HOPELESSNESS

[1] Ecclesiastes 12:8

[2] Philippians 4:8

CHAPTER ELEVEN:
LASTING GLOBAL SOLUTION TO DEFEAT AIDS

[1] Roddick, Founder and Co-Chair of The Body Shop. *Business the Ultimate Resource*, 2nd Edition. Page 1350

[2] Matthew 6: 22-23

CHAPTER TWELVE:
LIVING A LIFE OF MORAL EXCELLENCE FREE OF AIDS

[1] 2 Peter 1:5-7 NLT

[2] Isaiah 1:19 NIV

[3] Psalm 139:14

[4] Matthew 7:7

[5] Psalm 34:5 NLT

[6] Luke 11:28 NLT

[7] Jeremiah 33:3 NLT

[8] 1 John 4:19 NLT

[9] Deuteronomy 28:2 NLT

[10] See Psalm 1

[11] Proverbs 22:29 HCSB

[12] See Notes.

[13] See James 2:18 HCSB

[14] See Notes.

[15] Proverbs 23:7

[16] See Philippians 4:8

[17] 1 Samuel 2:9 KJV

[18] Romans 8:28

[19] Ecclesiastes 8:4 NLT

[20] Proverbs 12:24

[21] Ecclesiastes 9:10 NLT

[22] Matthew 16:18 NLT

[23] See Notes.

[24] Romans 8:19

[25] Proverbs 3:21-23 NLT

[26] Proverbs 3:13-16, 19 NLT

[27] Colossians 2:3 NLT

[28] Ephesians 3:20 KJV

[29] Genesis 49:25

[30] Psalm 2:7-8 NLT

[31] John 15:7 NLT

Chapter Thirteen:
Poverty, Corruption, and AIDS

[1] Romans 12:2

[2] Luke 12:15

[3] John 7:38

[4] See Philippians 4:13

[5] Isaiah 41:17 KJV

[6] Ephesians 5:3 NLT

[7] Psalm 34:10 NLT

[8] Proverbs 12:27

[9] Psalm 34:5 NLT

[10] See Proverbs 22:29

[11] 2 Timothy 1:12

[12] Proverbs 10:2 TLB

[13] Revelation 5:12

[14] See Psalm 1:3

[15] Proverbs 23:7

[16] Philippians 4:19

[17] See Colossians 2:14

[18] Proverbs 3:5 HCSB

CHAPTER FOURTEEN:
WORD OF KNOWLEDGE:
CAN GOD CALL YOU A MAN?

[1] Hosea 4:6

[2] Ezekiel 22:30

[3] John 8:32

[4] John 17:17 HCSB

[5] Psalm 138:2 NLT

[6] Psalm 37:37

[7] 1 Samuel 15:29

[8] Isaiah 5:13

[9] See 1 Peter 4:8 HCSB

[10] 2 Corinthians 3:5

[11] Jude 1:7 HCSB

[12] Psalm 72:7 NLT

[13] See Numbers 32:12

CHAPTER FIFTEEN:
DESTROYING THE YOKE OF HIV THROUGH PRAYER

[1] Matthew 19:26 NLT

[2] Acts 3:6

[3] 2 Kings 20:1 NLT (emphasis added)

[4] See Isaiah 53:4

[5] Psalm 55:22 NLT

[6] Acts 2:21

[7] Psalm 50:15

[8] Psalm 50:23

[9] See Psalm 144:15

[10] 2 Timothy 1:12

[11] Acts 20:32 KJV

SOURCES

Pastor E.A Adeboye: "Open Heavens" is a daily devotional guide to close fellowship with God. (http://www.rccgna.org/openheavens/). Pastor Adeboye has a Ph.D. in applied mathematics and is the general overseer of Redeemer's Ministries, a Christian elder statesman, a spiritual father to millions, and a devoted prophet dedicated to proclaiming the power of Christ. Redeemer's Ministries can be found at http://crm.rccgnet.org/.

Dr. David O. Oyedepo: *Maximize Destiny*. Dr. David Oyedepo is the author of *Maximize Destiny*, an outstanding book as well many other books. For more than two decades, has been part of the current charismatic movement. Prophet Oyedepo is the president of Living Faith Church Worldwide Inc.

Ayo Daniels: "Develop a Family Vision" (a message on family life on 26/10/08). Pastor Ayo Daniels is the senior pastor of outstanding and dynamic Lighthouse Christian Outreach Centre Lagos. He is an authority in the area of family life and an outstanding conference speaker. This message is available online at: www.lighthouseng.org

President Williams Jefferson Clinton: the forty-second president of the United States. After he left the White House, he launched William J. Clinton Foundation which focuses on worldwide issues that demand urgent action, solutions, and measurable results--global climate change, HIV/AIDS in the developing world, childhood obesity and economic opportunity in the United States, as well economic development in Africa and Latin America. Information on these programs can be found at www.clintonfoundation.org

Anita Roddick: Born in Sussex, England, in 1942, this British businesswoman is the Founder of the cosmetics phenomenon "The Body Shop": She received the United Nations' "Global 500" environmental award and the order of the British Empire (OBE). *Business the Ultimate Resource*, 2ⁿᵈ Edition, page 1350.

J.P. Morgan: (1837-1913). J.P.Morgan was one of the greatest financiers of his age. He was a remarkable businessman that helped avert a U.S. financial crisis in 1895: *Business the Ultimate Resource*, 2ⁿᵈ Edition, page 1334.

Rick Warren: *What on Earth Am I Here For.* Rick warren is the founding pastor of Saddleback Church in Lake Forest, California, one of America's largest and best known churches.

John C. Maxwell: *Think on These Things: A Meditation for Leaders* (Beacon Hill Press). John C. Maxwell speaks full-time for Injoy, an Atlanta based Christian leadership organization he founded. He is the author of more than a dozen books.

Dr. Myles Munroe: *The Principle and Power of Vision.* Dr. Myles Munroe is an international motivational speaker, best-selling author, lecturer, educator, and business consultant. He is the founder and president of Bahamas Faith Ministries International.

Relevant websites

www.livingwithoutaids.com

www.naca.gov.ng

www.unaids.org

www.cdc.gov

www.nmac.org

www.clintonfoundation.org

www.avert.org

www.dipoobisesan.com

Global HIV/AIDS estimates, end of 2008

The latest statistics of the global HIV and AIDS were published by UNAIDS in November 2009, and refer to the end of 2008.

	Estimate	Range
People living with HIV/AIDS in 2008	33.4 million	31.1-35.8 million
Adults living with HIV/AIDS in 2008	31.3 million	29.2-33.7 million
Women living with HIV/AIDS in 2008	15.7 million	14.2-17.2 million
Children living with HIV/AIDS in 2008	2.1 million	1.2-2.9 million
People newly infected with HIV in 2008	2.7 million	2.4-3.0 million
Children newly infected with HIV in 2008	0.43 million	0.24-0.61 million
AIDS deaths in 2008	2.0 million	1.7-2.4 million
Child AIDS deaths in 2008	0.28 million	0.15-0.41 million

More than 25 million people have died of AIDS since 1981. Africa has over 14 million AIDS orphans.

At the end of 2008, women accounted for 50% of all adults living with HIV worldwide.

In developing and transitional countries, 9.5 million people are in immediate need of life-saving AIDS drugs; of these, only 4 million (42%) are receiving the drugs.

Global trends

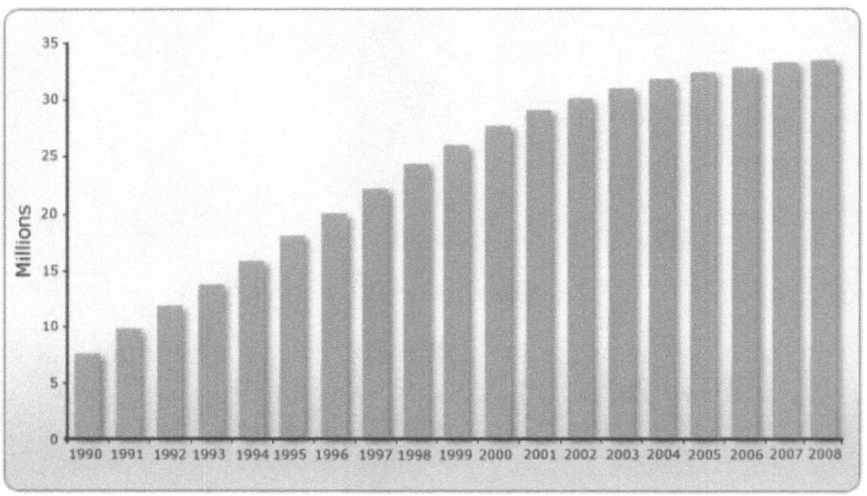

The number of people living with HIV has risen from around 8 million in 1990 to 33 million today, and is still growing. Around 67% of people living with HIV are in sub-Saharan Africa.

Regional statistics for HIV & AIDS, end of 2008

Region	Adults & children living with HIV/AIDS	Adults & children newly infected	Adult prevalence*	Deaths of adults & children
Sub-Saharan Africa	22.4 million	1.9 million	5.2%	1.4 million
North Africa & Middle East	310,000	35,000	0.2%	20,000
South and South-East Asia	3.8 million	280,000	0.3%	270,000
East Asia	850,000	75,000	<0.1%	59,000
Oceania	59,000	3900	0.3%	2,000
Latin America	2.0 million	170,000	0.6%	77,000
Caribbean	240,000	20,000	1.0%	12,000
Eastern Europe & Central Asia	1.5 million	110,000	0.7%	87,000
North America	1.4 million	55,000	0.4%	25,000
Western & Central Europe	850,000	30,000	0.3%	13,000
Global Total	33.4 million	2.7 million	0.8%	2.0 million

* Proportion of adults aged 15–49 who were living with HIV/AIDS

During 2008 more than two and a half million adults and children became infected with HIV (Human Immunodeficiency Virus), the virus that causes AIDS. By the end of the year, an estimated 33.4 million people worldwide were living with HIV/AIDS. The year also saw two million deaths from AIDS, despite recent improvements in access to antiretroviral treatment.

Notes

Adults are defined as men and women aged 15 or above, unless specified otherwise.

Children orphaned by AIDS are defined as people aged under 18 who are alive and have lost one or both parents to AIDS.

All the statistics on this page should be interpreted with caution because they are estimates.

Sources:

- UNAIDS (2009, November), "AIDS epidemic update"

ABOUT THE AUTHOR

Oladipo Obisesan is called into the ministry of intercession and head of The Ninth Hour, a dynamic and non-denominational prayer and intercessory ministry in Lagos, Nigeria, with a vision to raise generals for the kingdom of God. He attained leadership transformation through the outstanding ministries of Daystar Christian Centre, Lighthouse Christian Outreach Centre, and Word of Faith Bible Institute (WOFBI), all in Lagos, Nigeria.

He obtained a B.Sc degree in Economics with honors from the University of Lagos and had his mandatory National Youth Service Corps (NYSC) assignment as a Human Resource System Analyst with DHL International Nigeria Limited, Lagos. His day-to-day interactions with HIV/AIDS initiative groups ignited his passion to fight the challenges of this worldwide plague. He has since done extensive research on HIV/AIDS and related subjects, and now heads the Living without AIDS Mission.

Oladipo Obisesan is a registered member of the National Minority AIDS Council, Washington DC, USA, a member of the board of trustees for the Widows In Need Initiative, a volunteer member of God Sent Caring Mission, and President of Doorposts International Limited, a web solutions company.

He believes that everyone who is born of God has the desirable tools to attain success through diligence and prayerfulness. His philosophy of life is: "Success is discernible in prayer but attainable by action."

To find out more about
Oladipo Obisesan Ministries,
Visit us online at:

www.dipoobisesan.com

www.livingwithoutaids.com

Or send email to:

do@dipoobisesan.com

info@livingwithoutaids.com